Handbook of Veterinary Communication Skills

Edited by

Carol Gray, BVMS, MRCVS, PGCert Med Ed
Lecturer in Veterinary Communication Skills, University of Liverpool
Registered Practitioner, HE Academy, UK

Jenny Moffett, BVetMed (Hons), MSc, Dip Mar Comm
Director of Communications, Ross University School of Veterinary Medicine,
St. Kitts, West Indies

Foreword by

Dr Cindy L. Adams, PhD, MSW
Associate Professor of Veterinary Medicine-Clinical Communication
University of Calgary, Alberta, Canada

Introduction by

Dr Jane R. Shaw, DVM, PhD
Assistant Professor, Veterinary Communication, and Director, Argus Institute
James L. Voss Veterinary Teaching Hospital, College of Veterinary Medicine
and Biomedical Sciences
Colorado State University, USA

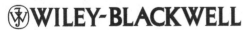

WILEY-BLACKWELL

A John Wiley & Sons, Ltd., Publication

Library of Congress Cataloging-in-Publication Data

Handbook of veterinary communication skills / edited by Carol Gray, Jenny Moffett ; foreword by Cindy L. Adams ; introduction by Jane R. Shaw.
    p. ; cm.
  Includes bibliographical references and index.
  ISBN 978-1-4051-5817-6 (pbk. : alk. paper)   1. Interpersonal communication.   2. Communication in medicine.   3. Veterinary medicine–Practice.   4. Veterinarians–Psychology.   I. Gray, Carol, BVMS.   II. Moffett, Jenny.
  [DNLM: 1. Communication.   2. Interpersonal Relations.   3. Veterinarians–ethics.   4. Veterinarians–psychology.   5. Veterinary Medicine.   SF 610.5 H236 2010]
  SF610.5.H364 2010
  636.089′0696–dc22

                                                                                              2009033003

A catalogue record for this book is available from the British Library.

Set in 9.5/12 pt Palatino by Aptara® Inc., New Delhi, India

1   2010

Contents

Contributors

David Bartram, BVetMed, DipM, MCIM, CDipAF, MRCVS
Veterinary Practitioner, Fareham, UK

**Susan Elizabeth Dawson, MBACP, PhD, MEd (SEN), BA (Hons), PGCE, Dip.
Couns, Cert Health Ed., MIFL**
Consultant Anthrozoologist Animal-Kind, Practising Grief Counsellor, Manchester, UK

Carol Gray, BVMS, MRCVS, PGCert Med Ed
LIVE Lecturer in Veterinary Communication Skills, University of Liverpool, UK

Martina A. Kinsella, BSc, ITEC Dip
Private Counsellor and Psychotherapist, Enniscorthy, Ireland

Mary Kirwan, RGN, BNS, MSc
Lecturer, School of Nursing, Dublin City University, Ireland

Geoff Little, MVB, MRCVS
Communications Training Associate at the Veterinary Defence Society, Knutsford, UK

Jenny Moffett, BVetMed, MSc
Director of Communications, Ross University School of Veterinary Medicine, St. Kitts, West Indies

Alan Radford, BSc, BVSc, PhD, MRCVS
Senior Lecturer in Small Animal Studies, University of Liverpool, UK

Foreword

In 1994, I was awarded a fellowship at the Ontario Veterinary College to study the effect of companion animal death on humans. At the time, awareness was increasing on preparing entry-level graduates to deal with this aspect of practice. End-of-life curricula varied between schools in terms of the time available to teach as well as the subject that was taught. The growing awareness of the need for effective communication with clients when their pets were close to death or deceased increased acceptance of the importance of communication in general.

When I graduated in 1998 and began my career in veterinary medicine, I was in a position to develop a research programme and communication curriculum that went beyond the issue of end of life to broader communication. This focus prepared graduates to deal with several issues in practice using a core skills set that varied depending on the context, urgency, and so on. At the time, only a smattering of veterinary schools in the United Kingdom and Australia were drawing attention to the importance of teaching communication in veterinary curricula. In general, traditional curricula paid little or no attention to communication. Practitioners communicated in a manner that was aimed at satisfying the veterinarian's need for data to solve patients' problems. The expansive literature in the medical field on the relationship between communication and outcomes of care was largely unknown to the veterinary profession. Good communication was considered a mechanism for making money, and any strategies for economic success were largely anecdotal rather than based on research evidence.

Over time, some influential studies revealed that the veterinary profession was lacking in terms of achieving results that included 'compliance' and employee and client satisfaction. The suggested strategy for ameliorating this situation was to teach students how to communicate, work in a team, and develop and manage a good business. Industry partners were starting to draw attention to the relationship between practice protocols such as 'compliance' and satisfaction; however, there was little awareness of how to distil communication into skills or ways to achieve the desired results.

A decade later, major changes have taken place and we are able to improve communication substantially. Veterinary schools worldwide have started to devote time to teaching communication and assessment. In addition, faculty members have begun to learn both communication skills and how to integrate communication teaching into courses on discipline and skills.

A great deal of communication research that has taken place in the medical field is applicable to veterinary medicine. Communication research into comparing the professions has also been carried out in veterinary medicine. Models for teaching communication have enabled veterinarians to develop more quickly than medical practitioners simply by adapting the models to our profession. We have been using textbooks from medicine to teach in veterinary medicine, and while this is useful to a point, there comes a time when the literature must reflect the context in which it will be applied.

To be successful, any textbook emphasizing communication in veterinary medicine needs to be practical and context specific. It needs to teach as well as convince the reader that communication is a necessary skill. The textbook needs to persuade the reader that communication is not 'psychobabble' but a core clinical skill that is no longer optional. Without skills and a commitment to continual learning, practice success and patient care are at risk. The *Handbook of Veterinary Communication Skills* meets all these requirements. The authors have done a superb job of describing communication skills and the major issues in the profession, including end-of-life situations using a skills-based approach. In addition, the handbook raises awareness of the various contexts in which practitioners need communication skills. The handbook examines a topic that has been largely untouched – self-care. So many tasks inherent to the profession, such as euthanizing animals, have previously been treated as inconsequential. The chapter on self-care now remedies this situation by promoting reflective practice to encourage the professional to engage in healthy coping strategies and take care of clients and colleagues in challenging aspects of practice.

Communication is poised to expand in our profession. *The Handbook of Veterinary Communication Skills* will provide teachers and students with a much-needed resource for both teaching and learning. All veterinary educators, students and veterinary professionals would benefit from reading this book.

Cindy L. Adams
Associate Professor of Veterinary Medicine-Clinical Communication
University of Calgary, Alberta, Canada

Acknowledgements

This book would not have been possible without the help of the following people. We thank them all very much.

Drs Jonathan Silverman, Suzanne Kurtz and Juliet Draper, for their unfailing support and advice on communication skills, and for allowing us to adapt the *Calgary–Cambridge observation guide* for use in veterinary medicine.

Dr Cindy L. Adams, from the University of Calgary, for her encouraging foreword and her enthusiasm for the project.

Dr Jane Shaw, from the University of Colorado, for her thoughtful introduction and words of wisdom.

Pete Wedderburn, Brayvet, Ireland, for his contribution to the chapter on 'Communicating with a wider audience'.

Everyone at the LIVE Centre for Excellence in Veterinary Education, the Royal Veterinary College, London, for their support and encouragement.

Introduction: The veterinarian–client–patient relationship

INTRODUCTION

To set the stage for the conversations that follow in this book, it is helpful to take an in-depth look at the veterinarian–client–patient relationship. This relationship serves as the foundation for all that we are trying to achieve in veterinary medicine, including satisfying the client, caring for the animal and promoting professional fulfilment. The dynamics of the veterinarian–client–patient relationship are complex with multiple dimensions to take into consideration.

As you read on:

1. Reflect on what approach meets your style. Often, we recognize a pattern that suits us most, is our dominant style and is our default pattern during times of stress. We are in our comfort zone in interacting with clients in this manner.
2. Take time to identify the relationship style preference of your clients. The overall goal is to demonstrate elasticity in your client communication so that you can tailor your approach to meet the client's needs and to enhance clinical outcomes. Frequently, communication challenges result from a mismatch in communication styles. Expanding your repertoire will enable you to meet the needs of a diverse clientele.
3. As an initial assessment, ask yourself, 'Who is doing the talking?' This is a simple litmus test for assessing your communication style. Are you doing all the talking, or are you creating space for the client to share their story and take an active role in the conversation? How much time do you spend listening to the client during the clinical interview?

A PARADIGM SHIFT

Recent societal changes have caused a paradigm shift in the veterinarian–client–patient relationship. Over the past decade, these changes have caused substantial transformation in

the veterinary profession. One of the major changes is the increasing recognition of the relationships that people may have with their companion animals (Blackwell 2001). When
asked about their relationship with their pets, 85% of pet owners reported that they viewed
their pets as family members (Brown & Silverman 1999). In conjunction with this, there is
a growing recognition that provision of veterinary services in a manner that acknowledges
the human–animal bond will lead to better outcomes for veterinary practices and their patients (Brown & Silverman 1999). Appreciating the impact of animal companionship on the
health and well-being of humans creates a new dimension in public health. Veterinary professionals' responsibilities have expanded to include the mental health and well-being of
their clients, as well as those of their clients' pets (Blackwell 2001).

With the advent of the internet, today's veterinary professionals are faced with educated
clients armed with questions and greater expectations. Veterinarians' responsibilities for
addressing questions and providing client education are increased. In an increasingly liti-
gious society, consumers are not forgiving of unprofessional services (Blackwell 2001). Most
complaints to regulatory bodies are related to poor communication and deficient interpersonal skills (Russell 1994), with breakdowns in communication being a major cause of client
dissatisfaction.

An adaptive response is integral to successfully addressing these societal and professional
changes. Given growing client expectations, the strong attachment between people and their
pets and increasing consumer knowledge demands a shift in communication style from the
traditional paternalistic approach to a collaborative partnership. Many clients are no longer
content with taking a passive role in their animal's health care and want to take an active
role in decision making on their pet's behalf.

VETERINARIAN–CLIENT–PATIENT RELATIONSHIP STYLES

The relationship dynamic between veterinarian and client is based on three criteria (Emanuel
and Emanuel 1992):

1. Who sets the agenda for the appointment (i.e. the veterinarian, the veterinarian and
   client in negotiation, or the client).
2. Importance placed on the client's values (i.e. the veterinary team assumes that the
   client's values are the same as the veterinarian's, the veterinary team explores the client's
   values with the client, or the veterinary team does not explore the client's values).
3. Functional role of the veterinary professional (i.e. guardian, advisor or consultant).

Paternalism

On the basis of these criteria, three veterinarian–client–patient relationship styles have been
described (Shaw et al. 2006). At one end of the relationship spectrum lies paternalism, characterized as a relationship in which the veterinary professional sets the agenda for the appointment, assumes that the client's values are the same as the veterinarian's, and takes on
the role of a guardian. Traditionally, paternalism is the most common approach to medical visits. Shaw et al. (2006) reported in veterinary medicine that 58% of all visits were

paternalistic, and, specifically, in 85% of problem visits veterinarians use a paternalistic approach. The topic of conversation is primarily biomedical in nature, focusing on the medical condition, diagnosis, treatment and prognosis (Shaw et al. 2006).

In a paternalistic relationship, the veterinary team does most of the talking and the client plays a passive role. This approach is often referred to as the 'data dump' and symbolized by a 'shot-put' (Silverman et al. 2005). Throwing a shot-put is unidirectional, the intent is on the delivery, the information to be delivered is large in mass and it is challenging to receive the message. Intuitively, it seems like this directive approach enhances efficiency and promotes time management. The challenge is that the agenda and subsequent diagnostic or treatment plan may not be shared between the veterinarian and client, compromising the ability to reach agreement, move forward and achieve full compliance. This could result in a roadblock, taking steps backward to recover and regain clients' understanding, commitment and trust.

Consumerism

At the opposite end of the spectrum lies consumerism, which is characterized by a reversal of the traditional power relationship between veterinarians and clients: the client sets the agenda for the appointment; the veterinary team does not explore the client's values; and the veterinary team plays the role of a technical consultant, providing information and services on the basis of the client's demands. The consumerist approach was not reported in veterinary visits and seems to be an infrequent approach (Shaw et al. 2006). While the paternalism model has been criticized for ignoring the client's perspective, the consumerism model errs in limiting the role of the veterinary team. The challenge in this situation is to engage with the client as a working partner and to build trust with the veterinary team to reach an agreement between the client and the veterinarian agendas.

Partnership

Between these two extremes is relationship-centred care, which represents a balance of power between veterinarians and clients and is based on mutuality (Tresolini & Pew-Fetzer Task Force 1994; Roter 2000). In the relationship-centred model, the relationship between veterinarians and clients is characterized by negotiation between partners, resulting in the creation of a joint venture, with the veterinarian taking on the role of advisor or counsellor. Respect for the client's perspective and interests and recognition of the role the animal plays in the life of the client are incorporated into all aspects of care. Shaw et al. (2006) reported that 42% of all veterinary visits were characterized as relationship centred, and specifically in 69% of wellness visits, veterinarians used a relationship-centred approach.

The conversation content of relationship-centred visits is broad including biomedical topics, lifestyle discussion of the pet's daily living activities (e.g. exercise regimen, environment, travel, diet and sleeping habits) and social interactions (e.g. personality or temperament, behaviour, human–animal interaction and animal–animal interactions) (Shaw et al. 2006).

In addition, a relationship-centred approach encompasses building rapport, establishing a partnership and encouraging clients' participation in the animal's care – all of which have the potential to enhance outcomes of veterinary care. This collaborative relationship is symbolized by a 'Frisbee' (Silverman et al. 2005). In playing Frisbee, the interaction is reciprocal, the intent is on dialogue, the delivery is airy, light and free. Small pieces of information are delivered at a time and the deliverer and the receiver adjust their message to stay on target. Intuitively, it seems like this facilitative approach takes more time; however, it was found that relationship-centred care appointments were shorter in length due to achieving common ground between the veterinary team and the client (Shaw et al. 2006).

Communication style has implications for the veterinary team, client and patient outcomes, based on research on the physician–patient communication that reported a positive relationship between aspects of relationship-centred care and patient satisfaction, physician satisfaction, patient health outcomes and a reduction in malpractice risk.

Specifically, the following principles of relationship-centred care are associated with significant outcomes:

1. Broadening the explanatory perspective of disease beyond the biomedical to include lifestyle and social factors is related to expanding the field of inquiry and improved diagnostic reasoning and accuracy (Silverman et al. 2005).
2. Building a strong relationship is associated with increased accuracy of data gathering (Silverman et al. 2005), patient satisfaction (Bertakis et al. 1991; Buller & Buller 1987; Hall & Dornan 1988) and physician satisfaction (Levinson et al. 1993; Roter et al. 1997).
3. Encouraging participation, negotiation and shared decision making promotes patient satisfaction (Bertakis et al. 1991; Buller & Buller 1987; Hall & Dornan 1988), adherence (DiMatteo et al. 1993) and improved health (Stewart 1995).

SHARED DECISION MAKING

Shared decision making is a key component of relationship-centred care. There is two-way exchange between the veterinarian and the client, identifying preferences and working towards consensus. An interactive approach (e.g. Frisbee) is promoted in giving information, in contrast to direct transmission (e.g. shot-put) (Silverman et al. 2005). With a direct transmission approach, the sender assumes that his or her responsibilities are complete once the message has been formulated and sent, whereas with an interactive approach, the interaction is considered complete only if the sender receives feedback about how the message was interpreted, whether it was understood, and what impact it had on the receiver.

Silverman et al. (2005) recommend using a 'chunk and check' method (e.g. Frisbee) when giving information, to avoid giving a one-sided speech and providing a large amount of information all at once (e.g. shot-put). The aim of this technique is to increase recall, understanding and commitment to plans. It consists of giving information in small pieces (i.e. chunks), followed by checking for understanding before proceeding further (i.e. check). In this manner, the information-giving process is responsive to the client's needs and provides an opportunity for the client to participate in the conversation, provide feedback or ask for clarification.

Taking the client's perspective into account and establishing mutual understanding and agreement encourage the client to fully participate in the discussion and commit to the diagnostic or treatment plan. This entails encouraging the client to contribute to the conversation (e.g. check) ('What questions do you have?'), picking up on client cues ('You seem a little hesitant about surgery'), asking for the client's suggestions ('What options have you and your husband discussed?') and checking for the client's understanding ('What will be the most difficult for you?'). Use open-ended inquiry to explore the client's perspective ('How do you feel Max is doing since the surgery?'); ascertain the client's thoughts ('What do you attribute to his good progress?'); and assess the client's starting point ('What do you know about the risks of arthritis?'). Extrapolating from medical communication outcomes-based studies, obtaining the client's expectations, thoughts, feelings and fears about the pet's health or illness enhances client participation in the appointment, with the potential to increase client satisfaction and adherence to veterinary recommendations (Stewart et al. 1995).

CONCLUSION

The questions posed at the beginning of this chapter included the following: 'Which relationship style reflects your approach?', 'What is your client's style?' and 'Who does the talking in your visits?' Given the answers to these questions, what steps would you like to take to expand your repertoire to meet the needs of your client? Flexibility in your approach is instrumental in meeting the diverse preferences of your clients. It seems appropriate to incorporate both paternalism and partnership in your toolbox and to interchange your pattern to meet that of your client. Matching the relationship between the veterinarian and the client enhances the potential of achieving significant clinical outcomes, including enhancing client satisfaction, improving patient health and, as a result, professional fulfilment.

REFERENCES

Bertakis KD, Roter DL, Putnam SM (1991) The relationship of physician medical interview style to patient satisfaction. *Journal of Family Practice* 32:175–181.

Blackwell MJ (2001) The 2001 Inverson Bell Symposium Keynote Address: Beyond philosophical differences: the future training of veterinarians. *Journal of Veterinary Medical Education* 28:148–152.

Brown JP, Silverman JD (1999) The current and future market for veterinarians and veterinary medical services in the United States. *Journal of the American Veterinary Medical Association* 215:161–183.

Buller MK, Buller DB (1987) Physicians' communication style and patient satisfaction. *Journal of Health and Social Behaviour* 28:375–388.

DiMatteo MR, Sherbourne CD, Hays RD (1993) Physicians' characteristics influence patient's adherence to medical treatments: results form the medical outcomes study. *Health Psychology* 12:93–102.

Emanuel EJ, Emanuel LJ (1992) Four models of the physician-patient relationship. *JAMA* 267:2221–2226.

Hall JA, Dornan MC (1988) Meta-analyses of satisfaction with medical care: description of research domain and analysis of overall satisfaction levels. *Social Science and Medicine* 27:637–644.

Levinson W, Stiles WB, Inui TS (1993) Physician frustration in communicating with patients. *Medical Care* 31:285–295.

Roter DL (2000) The enduring and evolving nature of the patient-physician relationship. *Patient Education and Counseling* 39:5–15.

Roter DL, Stewart M, Putnam SM (1997) Communication patterns of primary care physicians. *Journal of the American Veterinary Medical Association* 277:350–356.

Russell RL (1994) Preparing veterinary students with the interactive skills to effectively work with clients and staff. *Journal of Veterinary Medical Education* 21:40–43.

Shaw JR, Bonnett BN, Adams CL (2006) Veterinarian–client–patient communication patterns used during clinical appointments in companion animal practice. *Journal of the American Veterinary Medical Association* 228:714–721.

Silverman J, Kurtz SA, Draper J (2005) *Skills for Communicating with Patients*. Radcliffe Medical Press, Abingdon, UK.

Stewart MA (1995) Effective physician–patient communication and health outcomes: a review. *Canadian Medical Association Journal* 152:1423–1433.

Stewart M, Brown JB, Weston WW (1995) *Patient-Centered Medicine: Transforming the Clinical Method*. Sage, Thousand Oaks, CA.

Tresolini CP, Pew-Fetzer Task Force (1994) *Health Professions Education and Relationship-Centered Care: Report of the Pew-Fetzer Task Force on Advancing Psychosocial Education*. Pew Health Professions Commission, San Francisco, CA.

Basic communication skills

1

Mary Kirwan

Introduction

This chapter introduces the veterinary student and practitioner to the skills necessary for effective communication with clients (owners), animals, colleagues and support workers they meet on a daily basis. The importance of communication for all professionals is explored, making particular reference to health professionals. The skills required for successful communication are specified, with key terms relating to communication skills defined and some theories examined. Some of the models used to describe the communication process are outlined and their relevance is considered. A circular model that may be useful in the context of the veterinary consultation is proposed. The verbal and non-verbal aspects of communications are explored, and it is hoped that the reader will recognize the interdependence of both elements in communicating effectively. The ability to be able to ask effective questions is recognized and some general guidelines are offered. Following this, the importance of listening as a core element of communication is considered. Finally, the influence of the environment and culture on the communication process is considered.

BACKGROUND AND ORIGINS

The topic of communication and its importance in establishing and maintaining human contact can be traced back to the Bible. In the Old Testament story of the Tower of Babel, the builders of the Tower to the Heavens were punished and given different tongues. They were separated according to their language, with each group banished to a different land (Sundeen et al. 1998). Later in the New Testament, the story of Pentecost further illustrates the importance of communication: the disciples of Christ were given the 'gift' of tongues so that they could be understood by people of all languages (Sundeen et al. 1998). Neverthe-less, in the field of health care, such as medicine, nursing and physiotherapy, communication skills training is a relatively recent addition to curricula. The notion that *'talking isn't working'* was identified in nursing in a number of papers published in the early 1980s (Melia 1982). In relation to medicine, there is a view that effective medical consultations are still difficult to achieve despite the vast amount of communication literature (Roberts et al. 2003).

THE IMPORTANCE OF COMMUNICATION

'It is impossible not to communicate.' This idiom is often used by communication theorists (Laurent 2000). Communication helps us to learn about others and ourselves and is con-cerned with what is transmitted, how it is to be conveyed and what hinders or aids the process (Arnold & Underman-Boggs 2007). We are also reminded that interpersonal com-munication is vitally important to all caring professionals, and it is suggested that many of the problems associated with patient non-compliance could be avoided by improving the health professional's communication skills (Ley 1988). The lack of effective communication is a constant facet of complaints received by those dealing with complaints in health facili-ties (Roberts & Bucksey 2007). Hence, communication between health professionals and the client for whom they provide the care is important so that the client has a positive experience of the interaction (Roberts & Bucksey 2007).

In the field of medicine and nursing, communication has long been seen as a core com-petency for elucidating the patients' symptoms, problems and concerns and, according to recent research, an important clinical skill for ensuring health promotion, treatment and compliance (Ammentorp et al. 2007). Effective communication is largely considered to be a key factor in client satisfaction, compliance and recovery (Chant et al. 2002; Rider & Keefer 2006). The remark by Faulkner (1998), 'to be able to communicate effectively with others is at the heart of all patient care', is pertinent to any discussion on the importance of commu-nication. Studies have shown that when clients are involved in decision making they are more likely to adhere to the recommendations (Rainer et al. 2002). The statement written for nursing students and nurses is equally relevant to those in the veterinary profession. Inter-nationally, the teaching and assessing of interpersonal and communication skills are now accepted as an integral component of medical and related education programmes (Rider & Keefer 2006; Roberts et al. 2003).

Despite this increasing awareness of the importance of good communication in health care, a significant number of patients' complaints still relate to communication problems (Ammentorp et al. 2007). Misinformation, lack of information and lack of responsiveness are deemed to be at the forefront of such complaints in patients' satisfaction ratings (Ammentorp et al. 2007). The interface between communication skills and clinical skills is a common source of debate (Chant et al. 2002; Noble & Richardson 2006). In the medical literature, an example of the centrality of communication is illustrated in relation to cancer care in which the researchers predict that oncologists conduct between 150 000 and 200 000 consultations with patients and relatives during a 40-year clinical career (Noble & Richardson 2006).

It is imperative that health care providers develop an awareness of what exactly con-stitutes effective communication. Previous researchers and theorists have attempted to enumerate the skills required for effective communication. According to MacLeod Clark (1983), the following may be included:

- Observing and listening
- Reinforcing and encouraging
- Questioning
- Responding
- Giving information

Thus, to communicate is more than just the utterance of words but also the exchange of ideas and information between two or more people. In developing the Calgary–Cambridge framework to the medical interview, its authors established the importance of guidelines for doctors and medical students (Kurtz et al. 2003; Silverman et al. 1998). The veterinary consultation model is a version adapted for veterinary practitioners and students (Chapter 2). As in human medicine, communication in the veterinary consultation is goal-directed, time-limited and focused (Arnold & Underman-Boggs 2007).

DEFINITION OF KEY TERMS

Communication is the basic element of human interaction that allows people to establish, maintain and improve contact with others. It is the means by which a message is transmitted, how it is conveyed and what hinders or aids the process. There is inconsistency in the literature as to what constitutes a communication skill, if this skill is the same as an interpersonal skill and if it differs from a social skill (Chant et al. 2002). The literature would suggest that these terms are often used interchangeably (Chant et al. 2002; Hargie 2007). This poses difficulty in presenting an all-inclusive definition. This variant is particularly evident in the area of human resources. In the current era of competency requirements, many employers require candidates applying for a post to have high levels of social, interpersonal or communication skills.

Communication is the process of understanding and sharing meaning. Communication experts now appear to accept communication as a process with no beginning and no end (Hargie 2007; Wolvin & Coakley 1996). As such, it is continually occurring and constantly changing because no two interactions are the same (Wilson & Sabee 2003). This poses a difficulty if competence in the skill of communication is to be assessed (Hargie 2007). Some guidance in this area is provided in the work of Wilson and Sabee (2003), who suggested that competence is related to three qualities, namely knowledge, motivation and skill (Hargie 2007).

At a simple level, communication is the 'act of imparting of/or transmitting' and the word 'communicate' means 'to impart, to transmit, to be connected' (Simpson & Weiner 2005). For those in the helping professions, the latter 'to be connected' appears to be the most important. Communication skills are also associated with outcomes where the objective of the interaction is to achieve a particular outcome, as is generally the case in face-to-face interactions and professional consultations (McConnell 2004). Noticeably, some of the literature involving communication emphasizes the importance of the two-way function, the exchange of information between a sender and a receiver, while others stress the importance of understanding and feedback (Odell 1996).

Hargie (2007) proffers that communication emerges in childhood as a skilled performance and views interpersonal communication as a skill. He equates the acquisition of communication skills in the same way as gross or fine motor skills. Given that the basic elements of social skills are verbal and non-verbal behaviours, we begin to acquire a repertoire of social skills to a greater or lesser extent from infancy. In attempting to differentiate between social interactions and interpersonal communication, Hargie (2007) reviewed previous research and asserts that there are elements of commonality with social skills and other skills. He cites the six basic elements identified by previous studies (Michelson et al. 2007) as central to social skill acquisition:

1. Are learnt
2. Are composed of verbal and non-verbal behaviours
3. Entail appropriate initiation and responses
4. Maximize available rewards from other
5. Require appropriate timing and control of specific behaviours
6. Are influenced by prevailing contextual factors

Based on the assumption that these elements are central to the skill aspect, the following definition of social skills is presented (Hargie 2007):

> A process in which the individual implements a set of goal-directed, interrelated, situationally appropriate social behaviours which are learned and controlled.

In order to put this definition in context, the theoretical components of communication, which are believed to have a basis in three areas, are presented (Arnold & Underman-Boggs 2007):

1. The knowledge that underpins practice – includes theory from psychology and management.
2. The technical factors such as the skills used in practice, for example communication skills such as listening.
3. The creative component, the personal contribution of self.

This belief is resonant with the principles suggested by the enhanced Calgary–Cambridge framework (Kurtz et al. 2003), which clearly emphasizes these three elements, if in a slightly different order. The creative component (from self) and the technical skills are needed in initiating the interview and building the relationship, and providing structure to the process. The knowledge element is used in gathering information during physical examination and in explaining and planning the follow-on care. The creative element of self is important in closing the session and ensuring that the client/owner has received and understood the message(s) transmitted.

MODELS OF COMMUNICATION

Prior to examining models of communication, let us examine the elements involved in the communication process. These elements are the sender, the message and the receiver. The communication process is initiated by the sender who encodes the idea, feeling or thought to another person who receives the encoded message and begins the process of decoding the

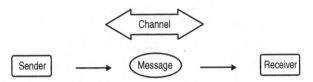

Figure 1.1   A basic linear model of communication.

content. Textbooks on communication illustrate this process as a model in an effort to highlight the core elements. A model can be described as 'a description or analogy used to help visualize something that cannot be directly observed' (Simpson & Weiner 2005). Figure 1.1 depicts this model as a linear process (Grover 2005). This shows a sender and a receiver and the channel through which the message is sent and received, such as the auditory channel.

A message is sent within a particular context; frequently, hidden messages are embedded in the verbal interaction (Ellis et al. 2006). A sender may intend to convey a particular thought or feeling; however, more than the exact message may be transmitted in the interaction. This is an important aspect of the communication process (Ellis et al. 2006). The receiver may grasp the message that was intended, in addition to other aspects. As the encounter continues, the sender and the receiver interact with each other, both modifying their responses in the light of the feedback from the other person (Ellis et al. 2006). The simple model outlined in Figure 1.1 fails to capture the important element of the two-way process of ongoing feedback. Attempts have been made to improve the model by adding a feedback loop (Figure 1.2). Adding the feedback loop recognizes the hidden messages conveyed in the non-verbal aspect of the process. A message is encoded by the sender and decoded by the receiver. Feedback is therefore an ongoing and two-way process. Therefore, the sender must transmit the message effectively for the receiver to interpret or decode the message (Grover 2005).

By using a circular model to illustrate, the communication process can be visualized as a cyclical process rather than a linear process. This conveys the idea of a process that is ongoing, changing and contingent on feedback. This is particularly useful when we examine possible barriers to communication later on. This circular model (Figure 1.3) depicts seven stages of the communication process and illustrates how some of the stages are subject to influences such as the appropriateness of the channel chosen.

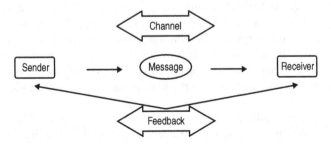

Figure 1.2   This model takes into account the feedback loop of the process. The message is encoded by the sender and decoded by the receiver. Feedback is, therefore, an ongoing and two-way process, as indicated by the arrows.

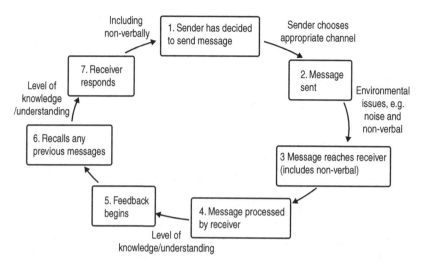

Figure 1.3 The circle represents the cyclical process of communication. The boxes represent the seven main stages in the communication process. Some of the stages are subject to influences such as the appropriateness of the channel chosen, environmental issues and the level of knowledge and understanding of the receiver.

What is the impact of supplementing a verbal message with written information or reducing noise in the environment in which the communication is taking place? It is advisable to have well-written information leaflets available to supplement oral communication as this will improve the process, as will locating a quiet area to reduce unnecessary noise. Additionally, the amount and depth of knowledge conveyed, or if the receiver understands the information, will determine whether or not the encounter is successful. The element of understanding is the key element when communication is defined (Odell 1996). Avoiding the use of jargon and unnecessary medical/veterinary terminology is an important consideration, as is allowing time for questions and answers. The circular model presented in Figure 1.3 is applicable to both verbal and non-verbal aspects of the communication, especially in the context of any veterinary consultation, as several messages are sent and received by the professional and the client/owner.

The concepts outlined in both the original Calgary–Cambridge model and the 2003 enhanced model are congruent with the notion of communication being a cyclical process, as outlined in Figure 1.3 (Kurtz et al. 2003; Silverman et al. 1998). This circle will be traversed several times during any veterinary consultation. Barriers to communication, and particularly to understanding the message being transmitted, can occur at any point in the circle. Some of these are the choice of channel, the appropriateness of the non-verbal cue, an awareness of the environment and ascertaining the level of knowledge and understanding of the client/owner.

Within a veterinary consultation, stage 1 involves the professional preparing for and initiating the process. The channel chosen and the words and tone used will set the scene for the consultation. As rapport develops, the process moves to stage 2, which involves considering environmental factors such as noise, comfort and non-verbal aspects of the client/animal and the veterinary professional. As the encounter progresses into stage 3, information gathering begins. The process of information gathering proceeds through stages 4 and 5, which will include the physical examination and past history of the animal being recalled (stage 6). It is important at this stage that there is mutual understanding so that explanations or treatment options are understood. As the relationship builds during the process, the consultation may come to a conclusion with a question-and-answer session to allow for clarification and the cycle starts again

VERBAL AND NON-VERBAL COMMUNICATION

Human communication is distinguished from other forms of communication by the use of the spoken word. The main channels of communication are the visual (seeing), the auditory (hearing) and the kinaesthetic (feeling), although all five senses (including smelling and tasting) can be used. Human forms of communication involve, to a greater or lesser extent, the use of these three channels. Throughout our childhood, adolescence and adulthood, we learn and unlearn how to see, observe, hear, listen, feel and react to situations.

Non-verbal communication

Communication refers not only to the content but also to the feelings and emotions conveyed in an interaction. Much of the meaning derived from communication comes from non-verbal cues. Non-verbal communication is defined as 'communication that involves all forms of communication other than the spoken word' (Ellis et al. 2006; Mirardi & Riley 1997; Roberts & Bucksey 2007). The old proverb that states 'actions speak louder than words' is very relevant to non-verbal aspects of an interaction between the veterinary professional and the client (Kurtz et al. 2003). There are many problems identified with the study of non-verbal communication such as the picking up of cues, which can be ambiguous, continuous, involve multiple channels and are culture-bound. The aspects of non-verbal communication discussed here cannot be considered in isolation from the other aspects of this chapter such as questioning skills, listening and the impact of culture on the communication process.

Functions of non-verbal communication

Non-verbal behaviours have a number of functions; they convey interpersonal attitude and emotional states of the sender or receiver. They can support or contradict the verbal communication, give the receiver cues about what is being communicated (in this case it is necessary to be aware that the person may tell us what they think we want to hear) and adds meaning to the verbal communication. They also substitute for language when speech is not possible (Argyle 1988; Arnold & Underman-Boggs 2007; Caris-Verhallen et al. 1999; Kagan & Evans 2001). Consequently, non-verbal behaviours have a regulatory function by allowing people to take turns, give and receive feedback and demonstrate attentiveness to the other person (Kagan & Evans 2001). Non-verbal communication can have five times the effect of verbal communication on a person's understanding of a message, compared with words spoken (Argyle 1988).

Components of non-verbal communication

Human communication, especially face-to-face communication, is largely non-verbal. Non-verbal communication is essential to convey acceptance, warmth, interest, love, respect and support and is essential to build rapport with other people. There is some variation in the communication literature concerning the number of components to be included when describing non-verbal communication. Variations of the list are common in many texts and include the following:

- Facial movements and expressions
- Gaze and eye contact
- Head movements
- Body movements and posture
- Proximity (interpersonal distance) and orientation
- Interpersonal touch
- Voice or paralinguistic features
- Personal appearance
- Environmental cues
- Time

Hargie (2007) uses just seven categories:

1. Kinesics
2. Paralanguage
3. Physical contact (touching)
4. Proxemics
5. The physical characteristics of people, such as colour or race
6. Artefacts and adornments, such as clothing and jewellery
7. The environment such as the setting where the communication takes place

There are ten aspects of non-verbal communication listed in the Calgary–Cambridge literature (Kurtz et al. 2003; Silverman et al. 1998), whilst the veterinary consultation model has shortened the list of examples to four key aspects: facial expression, eye contact, posture and position movement, and use of tone. By combining non-verbal behaviours, they can mean different things, and any movement can change the meaning. As these non-verbal components can replace, supplement or even contradict a verbal message, it is necessary to examine the main components with reference to their application in practice.

Facial movements and expressions

Facial expressions (Figure 1.4) provide a rich source of non-verbal information, especially in conveying emotion. Our faces provide our identity and, according to research (Knapp 2000), the face reveals six primary emotions: surprise, fear, anger, disgust, happiness and sadness. Facial expressions are therefore cues that help evaluate emotions and determine if the message was received appropriately (Grover 2005).

The various regions of the face can add further non-verbal information. These include the eyebrows, nose, cheek, forehead, mouth, eye region and movements, mouth region and tongue. Information about the primary emotions is conveyed in facial expressions, for example 'raised eyebrows', 'pouted lip' or even the simple smile. Therefore, through a very

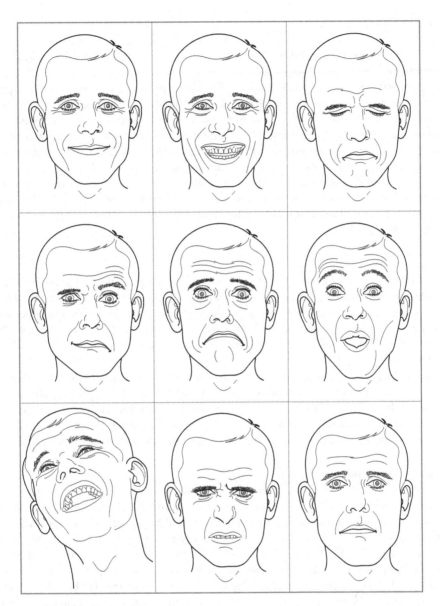

Figure 1.4   Facial expressions.

subtle change in facial muscles, it is possible to convey a range of emotions (Redmond 2000).

Information gleaned from facial expressions will tell you if the listener is pleased, puzzled or even annoyed by observing particularly the eyes and mouth area (Ellis et al. 2006). It is therefore very important that the verbal message is congruent with the non-verbal facial expression. Previous research undertaken suggested that the power of facial expressions far outweighs the power of the actual words used (Arnold & Underman-Boggs 2007).

Gaze and eye contact

Making eye contact is one of a number of skills known as attending skills. Attending behaviours let the other person know that you are focused on understanding and ready to listen (Arnold & Underman-Boggs 2007).

The appropriate use of eye contact is one of the most powerful cues we have for opening and maintaining communication (Sheldrick Ross & Dewdney 1998). Looking at the person with whom you are communicating is an indication of your desire to convey interest, empathy and warmth. Therefore, eye contact both regulates and synchronizes conversation.

Making eye contact should not be confused with staring or with a fixed eye gaze, which may be unnerving or may make the listener uncomfortable. Eye gaze is not merely a way of sending signals but also of receiving signals. Therefore, eye contact needs to be at a comfortable level for both the sender and the receiver. It is important to note that what accounts for appropriate eye gaze is bound up with culture and varies from culture to culture (Sheldrick Ross & Dewdney 1998).

Head movements

Head movements include gestures such as nodding, shaking or tossing the head (Kagan & Evans 2001). These movements can be used in a positive or negative way. In Western cultures, nodding suggests agreement whilst shaking the head means either disagreement or even disbelief. Appropriate head nods in the listening process will increase the speech duration of the client, a signal that you are interested and can encourage a fuller disclosure (Wolvin & Coakley 1996).

Gestures can replace speech and head nods are considered as attending behaviours in listening and are a positive indication to the speaker that their story is being listened to. As such, head nods are deemed to be a sign of a desire to be helpful in the interaction (Wolvin & Coakley 1996). Furthermore, people who use appropriate head nodding are considered to be more empathic, open and warm, all desirable attributives of a caring professional.

Body movements and posture

The way you sit or stand (Figure 1.5) can signal your mood or attitude to the other person (Sheldrick Ross & Dewdney 1998). A slumped posture can indicate boredom; a relaxed posture may suggest a person is calm and unnerved. A shifting posture may indicate unease or discomfort. It is essential to realize that your body posture can give the client a powerful message (Arnold & Underman-Boggs 2007). Whether you are sitting or standing, your body should be relaxed and the upper part of your body inclined slightly towards the client (Arnold & Underman-Boggs 2007). Matching or mirroring a posture may be used to indicate congruence and establish empathic rapport. Certain non-verbal skills can be used to visibly tune in to the client. These skills provide a way of identifying and remembering the type of behaviour that encourages effective listening (Metcalf 1998). The acronym SOLER is useful when applying the behaviours in practice (Egan 2002):

S   Sit squarely in relation to the client/owner
O   Maintain an open position
L   Lean slightly forward
E   Maintain appropriate eye contact
R   Relax

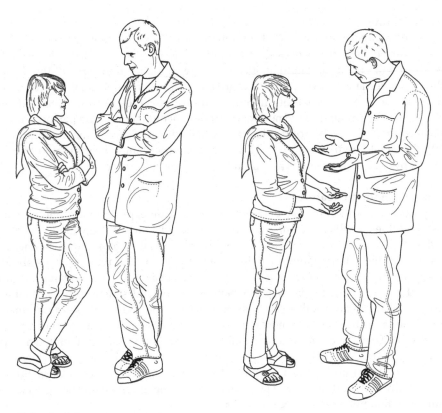

Figure 1.5 Body language.

These behaviours, however, may require adapting when communicating with different cultures (Egan 2002).

Proximity and orientation

Body zones were identified as far back as the 1950s when Hall identified four zones marking the areas of social interaction, namely intimate, personal, social and public (Wolvin & Coakley 1996). We all have an area that we consider our personal space and feel uncomfortable if this space is breached. The term 'proxemics' refers to the use of space in interpersonal relationships.

The intimate space is generally up to 45 cm (18 in.) and is reserved for intimate thoughts and feelings. The personal distance ranges from 45 to 120 cm (from 18 in. to 4 ft) and is used for less intense interpersonal exchanges. Both the intimate space and the personal space are influenced by age, sex and culture (Ellis et al. 2006; Wolvin & Coakley 1996). Professionals such as doctors and nurses frequently, in their professional capacity, have permission to invade this space. The same applies to vets if, for example, they need to get the assistance of an owner during a physical examination of an animal. The social distance ranges from 1.2 to 3.6 m (from 4 to 12 ft) and is generally the distance used for formal exchanges. Most interactions during a consultation happen in this space.

Interpersonal touch

Touch is a personal form of non-verbal communication. Touch is the very first way of communicating caring, i.e. touches between the mother and the baby (Fredriksson 1999). How we use touch will give information about the nature of the relationship and the degree of friendliness between the two people (Ellis et al. 2006). The use of appropriate touch is considered one of the non-verbal signals of a friendly and caring attitude (Argyle 1988; Fredriksson 1999). Messages such as affection, emotional support, encouragement and personal attention are conveyed through touch. Appropriate touch helps in creating and maintaining connection with the client (Fredriksson 1999). However, it is important to bear in mind that touch is governed by social norms and is also influenced by the cultural context.

Voice or paralinguistic features

'Paralinguistics' is the term used to describe the tone, volume, pitch, timbre and intonation, emphasis and fluency which accompanies speech (Sheldrick Ross & Dewdney 1998; Sully & Dallas 2006). Paralinguistic features accompany words to make up the true meaning. These features help in the interpretation of the message by giving the receiver clues about the sender's state of mind (Ellis et al. 2006). The tone of a speaker's voice can have a dramatic impact on the meaning of the message. A person's emotional state can directly influence the tone of voice. Sometimes this effect is unconscious and the words send one message while the tone sends the opposite message. Therefore, voice tone can be a cue to a person's emotional state. Fear, anger and grief are emotions conveyed through intonation and pitch of the voice. The paralinguistic aspects of an interaction are of particular importance when the other person is not visible, such as in telephone consultations. Hence, a warm voice can convey empathy and loud tones may be anxiety provoking and therefore act as a barrier to the communication process (Sully & Dallas 2006).

Personal appearance

Appearance plays a significant role in determining how a message sent or received is interpreted or understood. Hence, how one dresses and looks is a component of non-verbal communication. The dress code for an acceptable appearance can vary according to the immediate task and the culture. People form an impression of one another in anything from 20 seconds to a few minutes. The phrase 'a glance across a crowded room', usually used in relation to eye contact that occurs in romantic human relationships, is equally apt to describe this aspect of non-verbal communication.

The use of artefacts such as cosmetics, hair, accessories and possessions, such as make of car, provide prompts to the person's physical well-being, personality, social status, religion, culture and self-concept.

Environmental cues

The physical environment of the consultation influences the ability of both parties to communicate, and therefore to set up a successful communication one must attend to the environment (Arnold & Underman-Boggs 2007). The environmental context consists of those factors outside the people involved in the communication. It includes the physical factors such as location, the furnishings and their arrangement, as well as size of treatment room and waiting room, if relevant. One can arrange furniture to enhance or restrict the communication process. Also included are comforts such as heating, lighting and ventilation. Noise is an important facet when considering the environment (Redmond 2000). Radios, stereos and background noise from traffic are all relevant. Another aspect of this is the time of day that the consultation takes place. The environment may be either at the client's home or farm or in the consulting room. In either instance, the environment needs to be considered during the consultation. Including a relative or friend whom the client trusts can greatly increase the comfort of the client if the ensuing conversation is likely to produce anxiety (Arnold & Underman-Boggs 2007).

Time
Timing is fundamental to the success of the interaction. The professional may need to take account of the client's emotional readiness to accept a particular diagnosis or course of action. Remember that the client may be anxious or even angry at the event leading up to the consultation. Hence, planning the communication when the client is more receptive and able to participate is both time efficient and respectful of the client's needs (Arnold & Underman-Boggs 2007).

In summary, non-verbal communication is intrinsic to all messages sent and received during the communication process. A number of functions are identified including adding meaning to verbal communication, aiding feedback and sometimes substituting for verbal communication. Various taxonomies relating to aspects of non-verbal communication are available in the literature, and each aspect can influence the interaction positively and negatively for both parties in the interaction.

Verbal communication

Questioning skills

In our daily lives we all ask and answer many questions. Asking questions is a fundamental skill for all health professionals (Balzer-Riley 2000). This section examines some skills and practices that may make the process more effective. In Chapter 2, the structure of the veterinary consultation is dealt with in detail. The purpose here is to examine the skills required in a general way. The more effective you are at asking questions, the more time you will save (Balzer-Riley 2000).

It is possible to improve questioning skills by becoming aware of the different types of questions that can be asked. In addition, using a variety of questioning styles to elicit different types of information will improve the communication encounter. The main reason for asking questions is to obtain essential data that will assist in providing quality care for the client (Balzer-Riley 2000). One way of achieving quality care is to provide an equal opportunity to the client to ask, as well as answer, questions. This will allow the professional to clarify issues as well as explore and prescribe treatment options (Geist-Martin et al. 2003). It is important to consider that professional relationships can have an imbalance of power and asking questions can mark status differential between the professional and the client (Hargie 2007).

Functions of questions

A question is defined as 'any statement or non-verbal act that invites an answer' (Hargie 2007). The essential function of a question is to elicit a verbal (or, if not possible, a non-verbal) response from the other person. Questions can be used to open a conversation or to initiate social interaction (Kagan & Evans 2001). Other functions of questions include conveying interest, obtaining information, identification of problems, seeking clarification and ascertaining the extent of knowledge and understanding of the client (Hargie 2007; Kagan & Evans 2001). The type of question asked will influence the extent to which the various functions are fulfilled (Hargie 2007; Kagan & Evans 2001). Questions are also part of the listening process (detailed later in this chapter) when the question is used to encourage the client to continue or elaborate on the topic (Kagan & Evans 2001).

Types of questions

There are a number of different ways to classify types of questions. The main categories are either open or closed questions and the remainder are subgroups of these. This list represents some of the common classifications:

- Closed questions
- Open questions
- Reflective questions
- Probing questions
- Focused questions
- Leading questions

A closed question is used when there is only one answer such as 'yes' or 'no'. This type of question limits the explanation but can elicit important and concise information. Hence, this method is useful in eliciting facts (Kagan & Evans 2001). Closed questions make it easier for the interviewer (questioner) to control the talk, but conversely, may make the client feel threatened due to the limitations and restrictions imposed (Hargie 2007). Most closed questions will start with words such as 'do', 'is', 'did' and 'will'.

> Example: 'Did the tablets work OK?'
> Answer: 'Yes'

Open questions, in contrast, aim to get the client to tell a story. They invite the client to elaborate in a direction of their choosing (Balzer-Riley 2000). The idea of opening an interaction with an open question is recommended by many researchers and experts, and some suggest gradually reducing the level of openness by a process called *funnel sequence* (Hargie 2007). This approach provides clients with an opportunity to discuss the issues high on their agenda at the outset in a manner that comes naturally to them (Hargie 2007). It is important for the professional not to ask more than one question at a time, or move on to another topic, until the current topic is explored in adequate depth. In any interaction it is important to watch out for non-verbal as well as verbal responses. Open questions allow the client to describe their experiences, feelings and understanding of the issue under discussion (Sully & Dallas 2006). This approach can lead to pertinent, yet unexpected, information (Bradley & Edinberg 1986). Open questions usually start with words and phrases such as 'tell me ...', 'how would you ...', 'what seems to be ...' and 'which ...'

> Example: 'What seems to be the problem with Toby?'
> Answer: 'We were in the park and he ...'

This gives the listener an opportunity to follow up for more detail.

Reflective questions can be considered as a subdivision of either open or closed questions. This type of question is useful if it is necessary to soften the questioning process and also demonstrates to the client (speaker) that you are really listening to their story. Generally, reflection involves summarizing what the person said and therefore is similar to paraphrasing. In this instance, the client gets feedback and is aware that they have been listened to. It is important that this is done correctly as, if the message is changed, the communication may become ineffective.

Probing questions are used as a follow-up to the initial question to elicit the scope of information required (Hargie 2007). This allows in-depth exploration of a specific area. The ability to probe effectively is therefore at the core of effective questioning. A probe can follow on from either an open or closed question. It can take a great deal of sensitivity to determine how far to go in this line of questioning (Bradley & Edinberg 1986). Non-verbal cues are important – note that the client may tense up if uncomfortable with the line of questioning. There are different ways to approach probing depending on the purpose of the information that is being sought. For example, one may wish to seek clarification on a particular aspect or require the client to expand on a particular element. Accuracy probes can be used to check the correctness of what has been said. Probes can also take a non-verbal form such as raising the eyebrows (Hargie 2007).

A focused question is neither open nor closed but includes characteristics of both. The function of a focused question is to limit the area to which a client can respond but encourages more than a yes or no answer (Bradley & Edinberg 2007).

Leading questions, as the term suggests, lead to a predicted answer (Kagan & Evans 2001). Hence, the phrase 'putting words in your mouth' is used in this context. Leading questions can be subtle and encourage the acceptance of ideas, but may limit the possible replies (Kagan & Evans 2001). Using this format may imply that the person should respond in a particular way and so may limit the information that is transmitted.

In summary, it is important to remember that the same question can be used in different ways and in each circumstance a different response may be elicited. Knowing how and when to use different types of questions is useful in order to obtain essential data that will assist you in providing quality care for your client. Open questions encourage the client to open up and expand on the information. Closed questions are useful to close down an overly wordy or rambling response or encourage a more concise answer. Probing questions are useful for added detail. Reflective questions are useful to get the other person back on track. Leading questions have limited use in health and related professions. Critical to the success of questioning strategies is the use of attentive and active listening skills (O'Gara & Fairhurst 2004).

LISTENING

Any discussion on communication usually refers to the act of listening. To 'be listened to' is considered a core attribute in organizations, businesses and services and is a critical component of the communication process and the most effective communication technique (Hargie 2007; Sundeen et al. 1998; Wolvin & Coakley 1996). Expertise in the art of listening is essential when interacting with clients and colleagues (Metcalf 1998). Conversely, poor listening skills are cited in a large percentage of medical negligence cases and one of the main reasons why individuals take legal action against health care professionals (Rainer et al. 2002).

Listening and attending are cited as the two most important elements of therapeutic communication, with 'overtalking' the least productive (Burnard 1992). Listening and attending require hearing and understanding of both verbal and non-verbal cues such as eye contact and paralinguistic aspects of the message alluded to earlier in this chapter. Perception is closely related to listening as surrounding stimuli are taken into account when a message is being conveyed (Redmond 2000). Together, the art of listening and perceiving involves decoding or interpreting the message and gives information about whether the listener understands the information transmitted.

Defining listening

There are many definitions of listening, such as 'the selection and retention of aurally received data' (Weaver 2007), or 'the process by which spoken language is converted to meaning in the mind' (Hargie 2007). Some theorists regard listening as a purely auditory activity, a process that takes place 'when the human organism receives data aurally' (Hargie 2007; O'Gara & Fairhurst 2004). In making a distinction between hearing and listening, hearing is regarded as a physical activity while listening is a mental process. A more comprehensive definition by Wolvin and Coakley (1996) describes listening as 'the process of receiving, attending to, and assigning meaning to aural and visual stimuli'. This definition captures the complexity of listening and includes the three core elements of listening – receiving, attending and assigning meaning – as described in most communication texts.

Some literature describes the concept of listening with the addition of one of three prefixes: active, reflective and therapeutic (Fredriksson 1999). Additionally, these prefixes are used interchangeably, but the term 'therapeutic' is generally associated with helping relationships such as the relationship between a client and a health care professional.

In terms of interpersonal interaction, the emphasis is on the process by which spoken language is converted to meaning. Just as we see with our eyes but read with our brains, so we hear with our ears but listen with our brains. We do not need to learn how to hear, but we have to learn how to listen (Wolvin & Coakley 1996). In this sense, listening is not something that happens physically in the ears, but rather happens mentally between the ears and is a deliberate and active behaviour (Fredriksson 1999). Aural definitions of listening ignore the non-verbal cues emitted by the speaker during social interaction. Yet, such clues can have an important effect on the meaning of the communication to be conveyed during social interactions. As a result, listening is often conceived as encompassing both verbal and non-verbal messages.

Functions of listening

The goal of listening is to understand as fully as possible what the other person is trying to communicate. The functions of listening, in a health care context, can be summarized as follows (Metcalf 1998):

- To focus specifically upon the messages being communicated by another person
- To gain a full and accurate understanding of the other person's problems/issues
- To convey interest, concern and attention for the other person
- To encourage full, open and honest expression
- To develop a client-centred approach during the interaction

Successful communication is dependent on effective listening. This is crucial to satisfy the other person's goals and needs, as well as our own. Effective listening is a specific interpersonal skill that can be developed and practised in professional interactions. Earlier research on listening was conducted in academic institutions and the assumption was that college students learnt by reading textbooks and listening to lectures (Hargie 2007). More recent educational research, which focuses on student-centred education, emphasizes how listening and other communication skills are only part of the learning process. Contemporaneous research concludes that listening is more than just hearing and therefore is an active rather than a passive process (Stickley & Freshwater 2006).

Listening as a communication skill

Most communication textbooks consider listening a core communication skill, which would imply that it can be learnt and practised (Fredriksson 1999; Redmond 2000). It is important not to confuse the skill of conversation with the skill of listening as great talkers do not always make good listeners (Stickley & Freshwater 2006). Listening at the beginning of the consultation is fundamental to the success of the interaction. In medical practice, listening to the patients' story contributes to almost 85% of diagnosis without further examination or tests (Cocksedge & May 1999). Listening is integral to models of consultation (Kurtz et al. 2003; Silverman et al. 1998) as the professional gathers data on which to base diagnosis and treatment (Cocksedge & May 1999). The merit of picking up both verbal and non-verbal cues early in the consultation and the option to engage in 'the listening loop' (Cocksedge & May 1999) can contribute positively to the outcome for the client.

As already established, for communication to occur between individuals there must be both sending and receiving of signals from one person to the other. In order to respond appropriately to others, it is necessary to pay attention to the messages which they are sending and relate future responses to these messages, specifically to engage in active listening. This is clearly evident if we refer to the circular model of communication described in Figure 1.3.

Types of listening

Wolvin and Coakley (1996) have identified a number of different types of listening. They describe these as a hierarchy using a tree and its branches to illustrate how each type fits a particular purpose:

1. Discriminative listening is at the root of the tree where the listener attempts to distinguish auditory and visual stimuli. At this level, the listener is making a rapid assessment of the problem and it may be as simple as reading facial expressions.
2. Comprehensive listening is at the next level but located within the tree trunk. It occurs as one attempts to understand the message in order to recall a previous message or retain it for use later in the interaction. Some examples of comprehensive listening include attending lectures, listening to radio or watching news and current affairs on television. The emphasis is on listening for central facts, main ideas and critical themes in order to fully comprehend the messages being received. It is suggested that discriminative listening at the root of the tree and comprehensive listening as the trunk are the two

elements that support the other types, which form the branches of the tree and shape listening behaviours.

3. Therapeutic listening is one of the three branches when we listen to provide support, help and empathy to someone who has a need to talk and be understood by another person. In the context of this text, this is representative of the client/owner who presents for the veterinary consultation. Here, the listener demonstrates a willingness to attend to and attempt to understand the thoughts, beliefs and feelings of the client.

4. Critical listening is the second branch described, where the intention is to evaluate the purpose of the message. This is described as similar to meeting with sales people or listening to advertisements on the radio or TV. The speaker is trying to persuade the other person by attempting to influence attitudes, beliefs or actions. In this context, it is considered important to use the three other types described to make a critical judgement. Additionally, taking account of non-verbal as well as verbal messages is vital to the process.

5. Appreciative listening is the final branch. This form of listening requires that the listener distinguishes auditory and visual cues in the message, comprehends the message, processes the message and appreciates the content, so as to respond. Listening to music is an example of appreciative listening.

These types of listening can be linked to methods or used as the reasons to listen appropriately in a particular interaction, with each method having appropriate and inappropriate uses (Redmond 2000). Listening methods include listening objectively to gain information and achieve understanding (Redmond 2000). This compares with comprehensive listening described above (Wolvin & Coakley 1996). Redmond (2000) lists listening critically as a method and describes it as analysing and evaluating messages. This requires the listener to evaluate all information received by stepping back from the emotion and to use critical thinking before responding. Listening appreciatively, conversely, advises you to suspend objectivity and be open-minded and open to emotional reactions. Finally, listening personally is presented as a method of engaging the client; this is likened to the type of therapeutic listening described above (Redmond 2000).

Passive and active listening

Communication literature pertaining to health care generally considers listening to be either an active or a passive process. Many people share their ideas, concerns and feelings if sufficient encouragement is received. All this requires is a verbal or non-verbal cue 'mm', 'ah' or 'really', a smile, a nod of the head, a lean forward or a 'tell me more'. This is known as passive listening or minimal listening (Kagan & Evans 2001). Passive listening occurs when minimum acknowledgement to the other person is provided, but it is sufficient for that person to feel comfortable about talking.

Active listening is similar to therapeutic listening as described by Kagan and Evans (2001). Active listening occurs when an individual displays certain behaviours, which indicate that he or she is overtly paying attention to another person. In using this skill one is actively involved. It is sometimes called reflective listening as one reflects back the 'music of the message' received from the other person. Active listening requires the professional not only to hear but also to interpret the meaning and to give feedback (Arnold & Underman-Boggs

2007). Active listening requires the listener to ask questions, guide the flow of communication and seek clarification (Redmond 2000). An active listener shares responsibility with the speaker in order to reach understanding. Consequently, active listening is considered a dynamic, interactive process in which the listener suspends judgement (Arnold & Underman-Boggs 2007). Active listening involves giving time, attending to and observing behaviours, recognizing and responding to verbal and non-verbal cues and being aware of words and gestures including one's own. Additionally, in some incidences all that is required is to be comfortable with silence.

Metacommunication and listening

All messages include non-verbal instruction from the speaker. This is described as metacommunication or 'the third level' of communication (Sundeen et al. 1998). It is more than hearing someone speak. It involves being with the other person so that we give them time, attend to their non-verbal signals and listen to what they are saying. It includes telling the sender both verbally and non-verbally that you are interested (Arnold & Underman-Boggs 2007). The professional non-verbally communicates acceptance, interest and respect for the client/owner through eye contact, body posture and head nodding, and even by smiling. Listening is a basic principle to ensure that communication is congruent by endeavouring that all three levels of communication – verbal, non-verbal and metacommunication – are giving the same message (Sundeen et al. 1998).

Guidelines to improve listening

In order to consider how to improve listening skills, it is useful to reflect on the aspects of listening. There are four main aspects which need to be considered in relation to the process of listening. These are the characteristics associated with the listener, the speaker, the message and the environment. Communication moves in a circular manner, alternating between the speaker and the listener over the course of the interaction.

Characteristics associated with the speaker and the listener

The non-verbal aspects already discussed all impinge on the listening process. A number of positive correlations have been found between the characteristics of the listener and the ability to listen effectively. These include:

- *Linguistic aptitude*: Those with a wider vocabulary are better listeners.
- *Motivation*: If the listener is highly motivated, he or she will remember more of the information.
- *Organizational ability*: The ability to organize incoming information into appropriate categories facilitates listening. Good listeners can identify the key elements of the messages received.
- *Physical condition*: Listening ability deteriorates as fatigue increases, an important consideration for busy professionals and clients.

- *Disposition*: Introverts are usually better listeners than extroverts, as they are generally content to sit back and let the other person be the centre of attention.
- *Anxiety*: This reduces the ability to listen. If worried about self, animal or others, we do not listen carefully (Hargie & Dickson 2004).
- *Feedback*: When given appropriately, it assists with the art of listening.

Characteristics associated with the message

This refers to the ability to use clear, unambiguous language, avoiding unnecessary jargon and medical terminology. Each sentence used to convey a message must be structured to get one significant point across to the listener. Non-verbal behaviours are carried in all messages.

Silence

Silence used deliberately and carefully is a powerful listening response (Arnold & Underman-Boggs 2007). Sometimes, all that is required is to sit quietly with another person, using touch if appropriate. Silence, coupled with a relaxed approach, gives the client time to think. Some people are uncomfortable with silence and rush in very quickly with words or interrupt with words; however, the overuse of words has the effect of covering up feelings and may stop ideas emerging. Sometimes, to pay attention to what is not being said is as important as attending to the words spoken. Another use of silence is to emphasize important points that you want the client to reflect on.

Some listeners are uncomfortable with silence during their interaction and attempt to interrupt their silence by talking. Silence, as with many aspects of communication, is culture-bound and in some cultures it is viewed in a negative way (Ellis et al. 2006). Listeners can make use of silence in order to promote communication instead of being intimidated by it (Davidhizar & Newman Giger 1994).

Summary of listening

Listening is a core element of communication. Important components that are included in the definition of listening include receiving, attending to and assigning meaning to messages received aurally. The functions of listening relate nicely to the definition. The central aim is to understand, as fully as possible, what the other person is trying to communicate, and successful communication is dependent on effective listening. Listening is deemed a skill that can be learnt and practised and is integral to the veterinary consultation as this is the time that the professional gathers data on which to base diagnosis and treatment, as well as to build rapport with the client. Different taxonomies are used to classify listening; these aim to give guidance on the best approach to use in response to the circumstances of the consultation. Active or therapeutic listening requires the professional not only to hear but also to interpret the meaning and to give feedback. Metacommunication is linked to listening and includes verbal and non-verbal communication in addition to overtly making the speaker aware of the importance of their story. In order to improve the art of listening, it is necessary to take account of the characteristics of the listener, the speaker, the message and the environment in which the interaction is taking place. In some instances, it is appropriate to listen in silence and to allow appropriate time for the emotional aspects of the message.

THE CULTURAL CONTEXT OF COMMUNICATION

As the world is getting smaller and travel becoming easier, people from many different cultures interact in their daily lives. Veterinary practitioners and clients/owners are more likely to have cross-cultural professional interactions as individuals from other cultures settle and become part of the population. Culture has been defined as 'a learned set of shared interpretations about beliefs, values and norms that affect a relatively large group of people' (Redmond 2000). It is important, therefore, to consider the impact of culture on communication. References to culture have already been made in relation to several aspects of non-verbal communication. More recent research focuses on non-verbal cues within different cultures (Arasarathnam & Doerfel 2005). Non-verbal communication such as tone of voice, eye gaze, hand gestures, self-disclosure and use of touch are cited as areas that influence the interaction by the culture of the persons involved (Argyle 1988). This is a complex area; it requires time and understanding on the part of the veterinary professional and client (Ellis et al. 2006). An example of this may be gestures used in greeting such as embracing and kissing, whilst normal in some cultures, these are reserved for close family and special friends in an Irish or British context (Ellis et al. 2006). In some cultures, respect for other people is conveyed by avoiding eye contact, yet in other cultures this would show lack of interest. Emotional expression varies between cultures, and this may particularly impact on how the veterinary practitioner prioritizes telephone calls.

How individuals relate to each other is influenced by cultural heritage and values and beliefs (Sully & Dallas 2006). All cultures are composed of individuals of differing socioeconomic groups, educational background and ethnic and racial heritage (Sundeen et al. 1998). It is vital that individuals are not stereotyped according to their culture as differences within a culture can be as great as differences between cultures. A number of definitions of intercultural communication are provided in the literature, i.e. 'people of two different ethnic groups or cultures trying to communicate', or intercultural communication occurs when 'a message produced in one culture must be processed in another culture' (Arasarathnam & Doerfel 2005). Hence, cultural differences are more than national boundaries and include values and beliefs.

Rogers (2003) suggested that three principles – genuineness, warmth and empathy – alongside demonstrating unconditional positive regard are the cornerstones of effective interpersonal relations. Such an approach will give guidance in maintaining a person-centred approach, as advocated (Arasarathnam & Doerfel 2005; Rogers 2003). When communicating with individuals from other cultures, these principles offer a road map for the veterinary professional in facilitating intercultural dialogue and relations.

Clearly, no discussion on intercultural communication would be complete without reference to the use of different languages. Words have power because we respond to them (Redmond 2000). Therefore, it is necessary to choose words carefully when communicating with a person whose first language differs. Initially, pronouncing a client's name correctly will set the scene for the interaction. Some word meanings change with cultural groups and this can lead to misunderstanding of the message being communicated (Sundeen et al. 1998). Consequently, the professional needs to check understanding during any interaction.

Professionals are required to develop an awareness of the cultural context and adopt a flexible attitude when engaging with individuals from different cultures (Redmond 2000). It is important to establish the cultural norms when communicating with a client who appears to be anxious or stressed. Culture will predetermine behaviours that are outside the norm.

SUMMARY

References to the topic of communication date back to biblical times. The importance of communication in the heath care arena is firmly established; despite this, problems that relate to lack of communication and miscommunication still abound and remain the subject of much client dissatisfaction. This chapter attempts to present an all-encompassing definition of the skill of communication. There is agreement that communication is a process, which is ongoing. The definition of a social skill as presented by Hargie (2007) is a valuable and practical method of considering the communication skills required by professionals such as veterinary practitioners. The use of a model is a way of considering the central elements embedded in the communication process, the sender, the receiver, the message and the channel. The circular model attempts to depict the cyclical nature of the communication process and fits well with the veterinary model of consultation. Interpersonal communication encompasses both verbal and non-verbal aspects. Professionals need to attend to both aspects as non-verbal components can replace, supplement or even contradict a verbal message. Questioning skills and the selection of the most suitable type of question are central to good practice and the best use of valuable time. Listening is a core communication skill and central to the art and science of the caring practitioner. Finally, culture and the awareness of how a cultural heritage impacts on a consultation is a worthwhile attribute for the skilled veterinary professional.

REFERENCES

Ammentorp J, Sabroe S, Kofoed PE, Mainz J (2007) The effects of training in communication skills on medical doctors' and nurses' self-efficacy: a randomized controlled trial. *Patient Education and Counseling* 66(3):270–277.

Arasarathnam LA, Doerfel ML (2005) Intercultural communication competence: identifying key components from multicultural perspectives. *International Journal of Intercultural Relations* 29:137–163.

Argyle M (1988) *Bodily communication*, 2nd edn. Routledge, London.

Arnold E, Underman-Boggs K (2007) *Interpersonal Relationships: Professional Communication Skills for Nurses*, 5th edn. Saunders, St Louis, MO.

Balzer-Riley J (2000) *Communication in Nursing*, 4th edn. Mosby, St Louis, MO.

Bradley JC, Edinberg MA (1986) *Communication in the Nursing Context*, 2nd edn. Appleton-Century-Crofts, Norwalk, CT.

Burnard P (1992) *Counselling: A Guide to Practice in Nursing*. Butterworth-Heinemann, Oxford.

Caris-Verhallen WMCM, Kerkstra A, Bensing JM (1999) Non-verbal behaviour in nurse–elderly patient communication. *Journal of Advanced Nursing* 29(4):808–818.

Chant S, Jenkinson T, Randle J, Russell G, Webb C (2002) Communication skills: some problems in nursing education and practice. *Journal of Clinical Nursing* 11(1):12–21.

Cocksedge S, May C (1999) The listening loop: a model of choice about cues within primary care consultations. *Medical Education* 39:999–1005.

Davidhizar D, Newman Giger J (1994) When your patient is silent. *Journal of Advanced Nursing* 20:703–706.

Egan G (2002) *The Skilled Helper*, 7th edn. Brooks/Cole, Australia.

Ellis RB, Gates B, Kenworthy N (2006) *Interpersonal Communication in Nursing*, 2nd edn. Churchill Livingstone, Edinburgh.

Faulkner A (1998) *Effective Interaction with Patients*. Churchill Livingstone, New York.

Fredriksson L (1999) Modes of relating in a caring conversation: a research synthesis on presence, touch and listening. *Journal of Advanced Nursing* 30(5):1167–1176.

Geist-Martin P, Berlin Ray E, Sharf BF (2003) *Communicating Personal Cultural and Political Complexities*. Thomson Wadsworth, Belmont, CA.

Grover SM (2005) Shaping effective communication skills and therapeutic relationships at work: the foundation of collaboration. *American Association of Occupational Health Journal* 53(4):177–178.

Hargie O (2007) *The Handbook of Communication Skills*, 3rd edn. Routledge, London.

Hargie O, Dickson D (2004) *Skilled Interpersonal Communication: Research, Theory, and Practice*, 4th edn. Routledge, London.

Kagan C, Evans J (2001) *Professional Interpersonal Skills for Nurses*. Nelson Thornes, Cheltenham, UK.

Knapp ML (2000) Non-verbal behaviour and human interaction. In: Redmond MV (ed.), *Communication: Theories and Applications*. Houghton Mifflin, Boston.

Kurtz SM, Silverman JD, Draper J (2003) *Teaching and Learning Communication Skills in Medicine*, 2nd edn. Radcliffe Medical Press, Oxford.

Laurent CA (2000) Nursing theory for nursing leadership. *Journal of Nursing Management* 8: 83–87.

Ley P (1988) *Communication with Patients: Improving Patients' Satisfaction and Compliance*. Croom Helm, London.

Macleod Clark J (1983) Verbal communication in nursing. In: Faulkner A (ed.), *Recent Advances in Nursing 7: Communication*. Churchill-Livingstone, Edinburgh.

McConnell CR (2004) Interpersonal skills: what are they, how to improve them and how to apply them. *The Health Care Manager* 25(2):177–187.

Melia KM (1982) 'Tell it as it is': qualitative methodology and nursing research: understanding the student nurse's world. *Journal of Advanced Nursing* 7(4):327.

Metcalf C (1998) Stoma care: exploring the value of listening. *British Journal of Nursing* 7(6):311–318.

Michelson L, Wood R, Sugai D, Kadzin A (2007) In: Hargie O (ed.), *The Handbook of Communication Skills*, 3rd edn. Routledge, London, Part 1, Chapter 1, p. 13.

Mirardi HA, Riley MJ (1997) *Communication in Health Care: A Skills-Based Approach*. Butterworth-Heinemann, Oxford.

Noble LM, Richardson J (2006) Communication skills teaching: current needs. *The Clinical Teacher* 3(1): 23–28.

Odell A (1996) Communication theory and the shift handover report. *British Journal of Nursing* 5(21):1323–1326.

O'Gara PE, Fairhurst W (2004) Therapeutic communication part 2: strategies that can enhance the quality of the emergency care consultation. *Accident and Emergency Nursing* 12:201–207.

Rainer S, Beck MD, Daughtridge R, Sloane PD (2002) Physician–patient communication in the primary care office: a systematic review. *Journal of the American Board of Family Medicine* 15(1):25–38.

Redmond MV (2000) *Communication: Theories and Applications*. Houghton Mifflin, Boston.

Rider EA, Keefer CH (2006) Communication skills competencies: definitions and a teaching toolbox. *Medical Education* 40:624–629.

Roberts L, Bucksey SJ (2007) Communicating with patients: what happens in practice? *Physical Therapy* 87(5):586–594.

Roberts C, Wass V, Jones R, Sarangi S, Gillett A (2003) A discourse analysis study of 'good' and 'poor' communication in an OSCE: a proposed new framework for teaching students. *Medical Education* 37:192–201.

Rogers C (2003) *Client-Centered Therapy: Its Current Practice, Implications and Theory*. Constable, London.

Sheldrick Ross C, Dewdney P (1998) *Communicating Professionally*, 2nd edn. Library Association, London.

Silverman JD, Kurtz SM, Draper J (1998) *Skills for Communicating with Patients*. Radcliffe Medical Press, Oxford.

Simpson JA, Weiner ESC (eds) (2005) *Compact Oxford Dictionary*. Oxford University Press, Oxford.

Stickley T, Freshwater D (2006) The art of listening in the therapeutic relationship. *Mental Health Practice* 9(5):12–18.

Sully P, Dallas J (2006) *Essential Communication Skills for Nursing*. Elsevier Mosby, Edinburgh.

Sundeen SJ, Stuart GW, Rankin EAD, Cohen, SA (1998) *Nurse–Client Interaction: Implementing the Nursing Process*, 6th edn. Mosby, St Louis, MO.

Weaver C (2007) Human listening: process and behaviour. In: Hargie O (ed.), *The Handbook of Communication Skills*, 3rd edn. Routledge, London.

Wilson SR, Sabee CM (2003) Explicating communication competence as a theoretical term. In: Greene JO, Burleson BR (eds), *Handbook of Communication and Interactive Skills*. Lawrence Erlbaum, Mahwah, NJ.

Wolvin A, Coakley CW (1996) *Listening*, 5th edn. McGraw-Hill, Boston, p. 69.

A framework for the veterinary consultation

Alan Radford

Introduction

I am guessing that if you are reading this, you are an adult and you work in some part of the veterinary health care profession. That means you are at least 16 years old (and probably a lot older). However old you are, you will have had about the same number of years of developing your own communication skills. So with this wealth of experience, why should you read any further? Surely we know all there is to learn about communication, in both our private and professional lives? I suspect that the people who truly believe this statement will never actually read this chapter. For me there are two main reasons to carry on reading. Firstly, if we are honest, we all make mistakes in communication in our day-to-day lives. We even have an expression for some of these mistakes: it is that 'foot in the mouth' experience, when we realize we should not have said what we just did. More often, perhaps, it is that gut feeling when we realize that an interaction with someone has gone horribly wrong, but we cannot quite figure out why. And if we make mistakes in our personal communication, we surely do in our professional communication.

The second and main reason to keep reading is that not only are we imperfect communicators, but we can all improve. That is good news. As with all learning, we really have to want to learn, otherwise we are unlikely to get very far. But once we are motivated, we can then learn through experience. But how can we learn about our communication skills? In particular, how can we identify the good skills we use, and, just as importantly, how can we identify the things we could improve? At one level, you know if you get a thank-you card or a present that you must have done something right – but what? Conversely, we may get the occasional complaint, and nearly always that means there has been a breakdown in communication between our veterinary practice and clients – but where? The interaction between ourselves and our clients is highly complex and multi-faceted. Where can we start to learn about this process? The way we can learn most efficiently is by breaking such complex tasks down into their component parts.

For those of you who have ever been for a golf lesson, I suspect the following scenario will ring true. After first watching you hit a few balls, the golf professional systematically deconstructs your swing into its many component parts: the stance, the grip, the back swing, striking the ball and the follow-through. For those less impressed by a golfing analogy, imagine you went out for a meal one evening to a restaurant, and the next day a friend or colleague asks you what it was like. What we tend to do again is break the experience down into its parts. For this example that might be the venue, the starter, the main course, the pudding (my Yorkshire background peeking through there), the value for money and the quality of the service.

And what does this compartmentalization do? It puts things in order and it helps us not to miss things out. It helps us understand what was good about an experience or a task, and what could be improved upon. It allows for constructive criticism and promotes the learning experience.

So, how does this relate to the art of communication? Can a process as natural as communication be similarly deconstructed when you get to adulthood? Well, I guess you may not be surprised to hear that it can. Otherwise, this would be a very short chapter. What we will do in the rest of this chapter is learn about one framework or model that has been used to break down communication, in this context the medical consultation, into its component parts. Such models were originally developed by medical educationalists and are now widely used to train doctors and other professionals allied to medicine at all stages of their careers, from undergraduate to consultant, in the clinical skill that is the consultation process. More recently, these have been adapted and are being introduced into veterinary schools as a basis for teaching veterinary students. In this chapter we will learn about one of these models. It has a name, even though not a very catchy one: 'A guide to the veterinary consultation based on the Calgary–Cambridge observation guide'. The Calgary–Cambridge guide is one of the models that are widely used in medical education (Silverman et al. 2006). As we will see, the model breaks the consultation down into seven key parts: preparation, the opening, gathering information, giving information, providing structure, building a relationship and, finally, closing the consultation.

And who am I to take you through this process? Well, I was part of a group that developed the use of this model for veterinary training (Radford et al. 2006), and I have had the privilege to use it for almost 10 years, mostly with undergraduates. But none of that is important here. What is important is that I am someone who passionately believes that good communication is at the heart of best clinical practice. The learning experiences I remember, almost above all others from my time in veterinary school, relate to communications skills. How, when I watched a consultation by a now retired dermatologist, he always started by asking us what we thought about the clients and their reactions, rather than by asking about their animals' skin. And when I was 'seeing practice', how struck I was by the privileged position we have in the animal health business, and how, through communication, we can have either a very positive or a very negative impact on our clients. Seeing practice as a veterinary student is a wonderful thing; you rarely get to see other people consulting once you leave the veterinary school. Fundamentally, if we communicate well, then our clients will be happier, our patients will get well quicker and we will all enjoy our jobs more. So, let us take this wonderful and complex thing, the veterinary consultation, break it down into its component parts, and look at the skills that we use in each phase. Time does not permit much recourse to the scientific literature available in the medical field that underpins this and other models. Instead, I shall be appealing to your heart rather than your head. I will use some experiences from my personal time in practice to illustrate key points, but better still, I hope that you will come up with examples from your own practice.

A GUIDE TO THE VETERINARY CONSULTATION BASED ON THE CALGARY–CAMBRIDGE OBSERVATION GUIDE

The summarized version of the consultation guide is shown in Figure 2.1. Not the most beautiful of things on paper, is it? But let us briefly look at its structure, before we delve more deeply into its individual sections. The central spine of the model is simple and applies to all types of communication. We should prepare. We must open the communication (otherwise we would never talk to anyone), we must close the communication (otherwise we would be talking forever – I am sure we can all think of people who are good at doing that). In between, we give information and receive it. Communication is always a two-way process. The sidebars are where things get professionally more interesting, and they are arranged down the sides to reflect the fact they are happening throughout the consultation. We should build a professional relationship with our clients and we should structure the consultation. The clinical examination is represented as the jam in the consultation process. This model can be used for all types of veterinary consultation, whether our clients own one Yorkshire terrier, a horse or a herd of dairy cows. And it works for all staff involved in the work of the veterinary practice, whether you are a veterinarian, a nurse or one of the other people involved in client care. As often happens in chapters such as this, I will include some phrases in quotes to illustrate points. There are no prescriptive scripts. It is really important you always use phrases that you are comfortable with and suit your own communication style. Models such as this are not meant to turn us all into professional clones. They are tools that allow us to explore and improve our own consultation style, in a fashion that must be very personal to who we are as individuals.

PREPARATION

It is nice to feel special that you are important for who you are and not just the next in a long line of clients (Figure 2.2). And that is what preparation should allow us to do – to ensure that when we first meet our client, we are focused on them and their animals, and not on anything else, whether it is personal or professional.

Create a professional, safe and effective environment

Clearly, there are very practical issues here to do with the safe and secure handling of our patients. I speak as someone who had a patient escape me in my first job. The owner hunted the streets for several days, eventually finding his dog – he knew it would be with children. But what does our client need and expect? In small animal surgeries, the classic environment

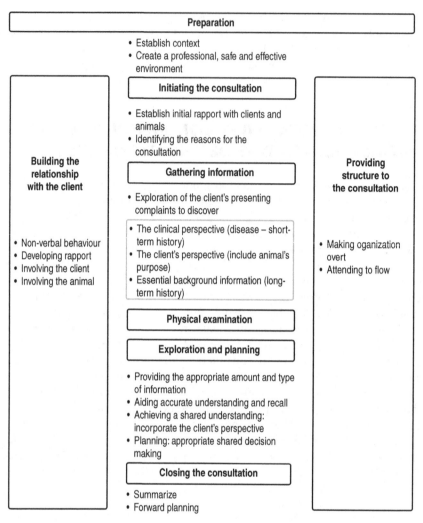

Figure 2.1 A guide to the veterinary consultation based on the Calgary–Cambridge observation guide.

is a fairly bare room with an examination table that divides the room into the client's half and the vet's half. This separation has been used for years to reinforce the professional status of the veterinarian. But what about chairs? Some less able people may well need to sit. One place where I used to locum had a low, broad window ledge and a chair, which allowed both me and the client to sit and talk, rather than having me towering over them. Even for the able-bodied, sitting creates an impression of dedicated time for communication, and may be appropriate, particularly where there is no need for a lengthy physical examination.

We also need to think here about how we appear. Whether we realize we do it or not, we often use a person's appearance to form our initial impression of them. This is not the place to be prescriptive, suffice to say we should have a professional appearance, appropriate to

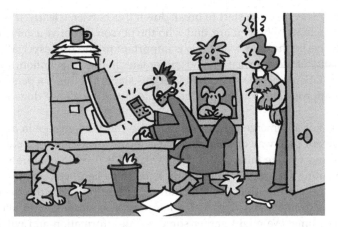

Figure 2.2   The busy veterinarian.

the animals we are seeing and in the environment in which we are going to be examining them (for more information on professional appearance, see Chapter 3).

Establish context

Whether it is in between clients in a busy small animal surgery, or during the trip out to visit a farm or a stable, there is always some time to prepare for the consultation. We should familiarize ourselves with the owner, the animal, the stated reason for the consult and any appropriate history. We can then start the medical process in our minds even before we meet the client. Another lecturer I remember, this time in equine studies, used to say when driving to the stable, 'switch Radio Two off and think about case'.

INITIATING THE CONSULTATION

This part of the consultation takes you from first meeting your client and patient to finding out why they have come to see you. There is a really important distinction to be made here. If you want your clients to be happy, then one of the most important things to discover is why they have come, not necessarily why you think they have come.

Establish initial rapport with clients and animals

How do you feel when you go and see the doctor or dentist? Are you at your relaxed and eloquent self? Almost definitely not. If you are anything like me, you are frequently nervous, and are concerned about the visit and what may be wrong with you or about to happen to you. This can make me inarticulate, often stumbling over my words. This whole feeling is reinforced by the fact that we rarely see the same professional these days. And the same is often true in veterinary practices. That is what many of our clients will be feeling like as they wait to see us – stressed, apprehensive and nervous – and this can create a barrier to efficient communication with you. And if you do not communicate well, you will diagnose less efficiently and your patient care will suffer.

There are many ways we can start to break down this barrier. Clearly, it is polite to have a round of introductions: who you are, and who the person is that you are consulting with. This may not always be the owner, and this is important to find out, especially in relation to assessing the quality of the information you gather later in the consultation, and in obtaining permission to treat. Some people shake hands at this stage, but this is a personal decision. It is nearly always appropriate to acknowledge the patient. After all, we do work in an animal welfare business.

Providing it is not an emergency consultation, we can then engage in a bit of idle 'chit chat'. We all have our own way of doing this – it is whatever we are most comfortable with. The English are said to love talking about the weather. I used to enquire whether people had been kept waiting for long. If you already know the client, you are in a great position to build on previous consultations by, for example, enquiring about the client's holiday. If you are lucky enough to be on a visit, then you can talk about the environment you are in. This is not wasted time. We might gather some useful information and will be starting to relax the client. It is also important to understand that people learn how to behave with each other right at the very beginning of a relationship, and this learnt behaviour is very hard to change. If you have an open and relaxed style with your clients from the beginning, then your client will quickly learn to be open and relaxed with you. Conversely, if you are closed at the beginning, you are likely to only get answers to the questions you ask.

Identifying the reason(s) for the consultation

A slight apparent tangent is coming up here. If I were to tell you I had just come back from a special holiday with my family and to ask you to find out about it, how would you do it? Stop and have a think for yourselves before you read on. Okay, most people start by asking really obvious questions. 'Where and when did you go?' is a good start. 'For how long did you go?' 'Did you stay in a hotel or was it self-catering?' 'Whom did you go with?' All these are examples of very sensible closed questions. But a far better way is to ask one open question, such as, 'Tell me about your holiday'. And this is a great way to start the clinical phase of the consultation. We all have our own phrases and it is important to use one you are comfortable with. 'What can we do for Buster today?', or 'What seems to be the problem?' If we do take this more open route of questioning then this next bit is really important. If we ask the open question, then we should shut up and listen. There is good evidence that whilst many medical professionals start with an open question, they interrupt after approximately 18 seconds and start focusing on their agenda (Beckman & Frankel 1984). What this does is educate the client to move into a closed mode, and only respond to questions they are directly asked. It is much better to let them finish. Again, the evidence is clear. Very few people talk for more than 30 seconds in response to this first open question. And if we listen, we will gather a large part of the clinical history, and probably a lot more than if we had just asked closed questions.

So, you have asked your open question and you have shut up and listened. The client will likely tell you about their major concern. But what about all their other concerns? Most people are worried about more than one thing. One easy way to address these other concerns is to acknowledge the owner's initial (or major) presenting complaint and then to repeat the open question. So, for example, 'apart from Bonnie's vomiting, is there anything else you are worried about?' And again, we shut up and listen. Essentially, we can repeat this loop until the owner says that that is everything. This is known as summarizing and is a useful technique at each stage of the consultation. There should then be no nasty surprises at the end of the consultation. A good example of this is a pyometra in a bitch. The owner may respond to our initial open question by telling us that Bonnie is off colour and vomiting. This might initially lead us to have a gastroenteric diagnosis at the top of our list. If, however, we do ask, 'Is there anything else?', then they may tell us that Bonnie is also drinking a lot. This is a very rapid and efficient way of setting the scene for the rest of the consultation, and critically allows the owner to share all their concerns. And remember, owners' concerns need not necessarily just relate directly to their animal's medical condition. An equally valid concern is the farmer who is desperately worried about the financial implications of your visit, and such concerns also need to be addressed during the consultation. All we have to do is listen. Using this method, even our first year students can collect good histories for fairly complicated conditions, without ever having heard of the actual condition in question.

GATHERING INFORMATION

Having already established all the owners' concerns through this repetitive loop of open questioning and listening, we can now use our clinical knowledge to finish collecting the history.

The order in which this is done is not really important, but this is one time when it is nice to explain to the owners how we would like to proceed with the consultation, by making the structure of the consultation overt. For example, 'I am going to start by asking some general questions about your farm and your herd, and then I will come back to your concern about the number of lame cows you have ... is that okay?'

The clinical perspective (disease – short-term history)

This is where we drill down on the specifics of the presenting complaint. It is the duration, severity, frequency, progression and response to any treatments given. And it needs to be done for all presenting complaints. It need not (and should not) be a big, long list of closed questions. We can still start with an open question style and fill in the critical gaps with more closed questions.

Essential background information (long-term history)

Much of this may be available to you through your previous experience of the client or from the records. However, these are not always correct. Important information includes signalment (age, sex, breed), how long the animal has been in the owner's possession, management (housing, feeding, use), routine procedures (vaccinations, worming, surgery), past medical and surgical history including medications, and where appropriate, the health status of in-contact animals including the owner and their family. To avoid the possibility of asking a lot of questions that some owners may feel you should know the answer to, it is sometimes useful to impress them with the knowledge you have gleaned from their records during the preparation phase, and then ask them if this is correct. For example, 'I have not met you before, but according to my records, Rover is 6 months old, you bought him as a puppy from the breeder, he has not been castrated, but we did vaccinate him here when he was 3 months old – is that correct?' This can inspire confidence in you and your practice (unless, of course, the owner comes back and says, 'No, this is Bonnie, she is 12 years old, was neutered when she was 1 year old and has never been vaccinated'). The only way it could be any worse is if Rover was euthanized in the practice last year, something you had clearly overlooked. There is no substitute for good records; we just need to make the time to read them.

The client's perspective (including animal's purpose)

This is a really important part of the consultation and reflects the wide diversity of our clients, their previous experiences and their relationship to our patient. There is the clear stereotype of farmers being motivated by money rather than welfare, and small animal owners being motivated by length of life and less about money. But what about the pet goat and the racing greyhound? Whilst some people do not worry much, others may be very worried. Consider the owner whose horse probably has mild spasmodic colic, but whose previous horse died of torsion of the large colon, or the owner of the dog with lymphoma, whose partner recently died of leukaemia. This is sometimes referred to as 'emotional baggage'. Understanding these concerns is critical to the treatment of our patients. Whilst we may feel our concerns are for the animal, the animal is treated via its owner, and our job in the veterinary profession is to help our owners make informed decisions about the treatment of their animals. For some of us, this can be extremely scary stuff because it exposes us to things that are personal. It may uncover emotions, and we are likely to need to show a good deal of empathy. (For more information on dealing with clients' emotions, please see Chapter 4).

GIVING INFORMATION – EXPLANATION AND PLANNING

You have taken your history and finished the physical examination, and come to your professional conclusion. It is now time to explain everything to the owner. Sometimes this may be very simple, but more often than not, we need to impart a lot of complicated information. And it is not sufficient just to tell our owners. It is also our duty to help them to understand and recall, so that they can make not just a decision, but a truly informed decision. In times gone by, receivers of medical care were told what to do, the advice of the medical professional being gospel. However, those days have now gone, and decision making is generally much more of a partnership between you and your clients that necessitates imparting all the necessary information to allow the client to balance the advantages and disadvantages of each treatment option. In those cases where clients truly want you to make decisions for them, it is still necessary to carefully explain the reasoning for choosing a preferred option, and the reasons for ignoring other options.

Providing the appropriate amount and type of information

It may be necessary before undertaking complex explanations to find out what a client's current knowledge base is. I am sure we have all had to give information to medical doctors about their animals. When I go to the doctor I usually tell them I am a vet. For me this means I can have a more meaningful discussion about my reason for visiting. It may also be that some of our clients have had experience of a particular condition before. It is certainly increasingly true that many clients have 'Googled' and 'wiki'd' before they get to you, so are variably informed or misinformed. Deciding how much information to tell someone requires careful judgment, and is best decided in consultation with the owner. A simple place to start can be by asking the owner, 'Have you any experience of this condition?' This allows the owner to say no, without feeling foolish.

Aiding accurate understanding and recall

There is no point telling a client anything if they cannot use the information or remember it. That is a waste of your time, belittles the client and has a negative impact on the relationship between the client and the practice. Suppose a car driver pulls up next to you and says they are running out of petrol and could you tell them the way to the nearest petrol station. How do you do it? Not only must you tell them the directions, you must help them remember. Common skills you can use are to break the information down into bits and explain this to them. 'First I'll tell you how to get to the cathedral, and then I will explain how to get from there to the garage.' You could also ask them if they know how to get to a well-known landmark closer to the petrol station. If they do, then there is no need to explain the whole thing to them, leaving them free to concentrate on the bit they really need to remember. You could ask them to go over the route afterwards to see if they got it right. This is actually something a lot of people do for themselves. 'Okay. Can I just check I have got this right ...'. All these skills apply to complex medical information. We should break the information down into small chunks, we should prioritize it, we should use repetition and summaries to reinforce the information, and avoid using overly complicated words if they are unnecessary. Of course, we may not need to rely only on verbal communication: they say pictures paint a thousand words, so we should make use of them when we can. There is now also an increasing number of models, professional artwork and owner leaflets that can all be used to aid understanding.

Achieving a shared understanding: incorporate the client's perspective

Although this part of the consultation is supposed to be about giving the client the information, it should not be a one-way process. We must relate our explanation to the owner's presenting complaints, and make sure we have answered all their concerns. For example, in the earlier example of the pyometra, we may say, 'Does that help you to understand why Bonnie is not only vomiting, but also drinking a lot?' We should give our clients the opportunity to ask clarifying questions, and even if they do not, we should be alert to their non-verbal communication for evidence that they do not understand. It is our professional responsibility not just to give the right information but to make sure clients have understood it, so that then, and only then, can they make an informed decision.

We must also realize that telling people a lot of information can have a profound emotional impact on them and we should acknowledge this. It is all part of showing empathy: 'I'm sorry to give you all this information. I realize it is a lot to take in. Is there anything you want to ask me?'; 'Listen, I can see this is very upsetting for you, just take your time'. By using phrases such as these, we show we understand as well as provide a practical solution to our client's predicament.

Planning: appropriate shared decision making

We have to remember that, at the end of the day, we are aiming to give clients information so that they can make an informed decision about what is best for the treatment of their animals.

Therefore, we must encourage the client to contribute their thoughts, ideas, suggestions and preferences so that ultimately we can negotiate a mutually acceptable plan. Treatment plans are about offering choices rather than giving directives. For more information on decision making, please see Chapter 3.

PROVIDING STRUCTURE TO THE CONSULTATION

This is one of my favourite parts of the consultation model. It is such a simple thing, but it can help all the parties in the consultation enormously. It ensures we do not miss things out, which is especially important as clients do not know the order we are planning to do things in, and it helps the client know where they are in the process.

Attending to flow and making organization overt

This is our professional responsibility. It is about making sure we stick to time whenever possible. And it is also about structuring the consultation in a logical order, one that satisfies the needs of both the client and the vet. But more than this, it is about explaining to owners how the consultation will be structured. This is sometimes referred to as 'signposting'. If you structure the consultation well and explain that structure, it puts clients at ease and helps everyone make best use of the limited time available. As an example, our family recently made use of the UK's NHS maternity services, and we were very impressed with the level of care we received. But there was one strange day when we went for a routine check-up, one of our first. We did not know how the system worked, nor did we really know what would happen to us. We were passed from health care professional to health care professional, from administrators, to care assistants, to nurses, to junior doctors and eventually to the consultant. At no stage in the process did we know what or who was coming next. It was quite unnerving and meant we probably asked all the right questions but at the wrong time to the wrong person. If someone had simply explained the order of the process, it would have put us much more at ease, and ultimately made the process more efficient both for us and for the medical professionals we saw that day.

We have come across this signposting a little already. It is really good if we can explain to owners the order in which we are going to take the history, and we can say to owners that we are going to give them lots of information, but there will be plenty of time at the end to ask any questions. Or we can even give them the 'permission' to interrupt at anytime. Someone once told me that a good way to give a lecture is first, to tell them what you are going to tell them, then to tell them, and finally, tell them you have told them. This same principle probably also works in the consultation.

BUILDING A RELATIONSHIP

This is the part of the consultation process that can often be overlooked, yet it is probably one of the most important. It uses a lot of those skills that we develop throughout our lives. With some thought, however, we can modify our behaviour to ensure a better clinical outcome.

Non-verbal behaviour

We tend to think of communication as what is said or perhaps written. But a lot is also communicated from our perception of each other's body language. There is a really simple exercise you can do here. Ask a friend or colleague to listen to you for 2 minutes while you talk about yourself. Then, swap round and listen to them doing the same. The only rule is that the listener cannot talk. When you have finished, ask yourselves, what did the listener do that made it easier for you to talk? And conversely, was there anything the listener did that put the speaker off? If you do this simple exercise, you will learn a lot about listening . . . and probably find out a few surprising things about the speaker too.

Eye contact is very important. It is probably okay for us to look away sometimes when we are speaking. When we are listening, however, eye contact is critical. If a client seeks eye contact with us whilst they are talking, but we are looking out of the window, the clear message the client will get is that we are bored. It is almost impossible to look at a watch whilst listening without at the same time conveying boredom. As well as eye contact during listening, we can support a speaker by nodding, and saying encouraging things, such as 'I see' or 'that's helpful', or even those funny little words that we all use that are in no dictionary and are really hard to spell such as 'mmm' and 'aha'. Laughing at the appropriate time is really supportive, but smiling at the wrong time can be really off-putting. Our posture is important as well and will be affected by the room set-up. People often ask about the use of a computer or taking notes. It is likely that these are best left to when the client has gone, but if we feel it necessary, then all we have to do is ask the client's permission.

This is probably the best time in this chapter to think about physical contact (Figure 2.3). As veterinary professionals, should we touch our clients? We spoke earlier about shaking hands, but what I am thinking about here is how to comfort an emotional client, and in particular should you hug them or place a reassuring hand on their shoulder, arm, back, hand or knee? Of all the sections in this book, if not this chapter, how you comfort upset clients has to be matched to your own personality and governed by what you are comfortable with. There are no rules. However, some people do say you should never touch a client

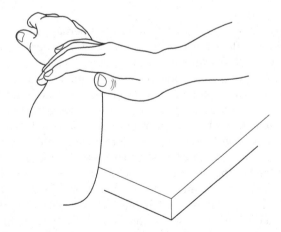

Figure 2.3   Physical contact.

for fear of being sued. Whilst I see the logic, I do not like rules that are made up to try and prevent what are extremely rare occurrences, being applied to everyday practice. Nor am I going to say the converse – you must touch an upset client. That is clearly stupid. However, you may feel with a particular client that some physical contact at a time of high emotion is appropriate. Clearly, it can be easier to interact this way with a client you have known for some time. But, even for someone you have met for the first time, a hand rested on the upper forearm can be appropriate. Done well, not only will this help convey your empathy, but it can help the client at a difficult time, when sometimes there are no words to be said. And also, I firmly believe that for some people, and here I am thinking about you, the veterinary professional, such emotional consultations can offer the greatest professional satisfaction. Some of the most satisfying consultations can be those where we have been involved in the life and death of an animal, sometimes over several years, have got to know the client, and been able to, in some small way, help them through the death of their animal, especially if this was a euthanasia. So, to summarize physical contact, there are no rules, and above all stay true to yourself. It is clearly not compulsory, but equally I do not think it should be banned, and where appropriate can have a positive impact on clients and vets alike.

When we communicate, we do so not just by our words but by our body language. What is really amazing is that when, as listeners, we receive conflicting information (such as when words say one thing, but body language says something else), we tend to pay more attention to the body language. So, if we are listening to someone and saying all the right things, but our body language says we are bored and disinterested, that is the impression our clients are likely to go away with. This highlights the power of our body language. To summarize this section, some people think of listening as a passive process. But it is not, or at least it should not be. Active listening promotes the gathering of information, and that is what a large part of a good consultation is about (see Chapter 1 for more information on active listening).

Developing rapport

Rapport means a harmonious relationship. It implies a connection between people, and moves the consultation away from just the exchange of facts, to a true professional relationship. One definition for rapport is camaraderie. I like that. It suggests the vet and the client are in this together. It puts us on the same side.

There are many ways to achieve this camaraderie but perhaps the most important is empathy. In the medical consultation it has been described as 'appreciation of the patient's emotions and expression of that awareness to the patient' (Stepien & Baernstein 2006). Empathy therefore implies not only a personal recognition of how a client may be feeling but letting the client know of our awareness. This can be summarized by the simple phrase 'I can see you are very upset'. I suspect empathy is where many of the boxes of chocolates and thank you cards come from. We can show empathy for lots of things. For the difficult financial market our clients may be working in. For the difficult decision we have just asked them to make. For the bad news we have just given them. For the size of the bill they have just received. Even for the fact they are angry. If we show empathy, research in medical practice suggests that our clients will be more satisfied and more likely to adhere to treatments (Haslam 2007). Unfortunately, other research in medicine suggests that for many physicians, empathy becomes eroded over time. I guess this is something many of us can empathize with. But it is something to be guarded against.

However, simply showing empathy is not enough. We must also, wherever possible, provide our clients with the support they need to get through what are often very difficult situations. These can be very practical offers of help such as an advice leaflet, or a suggestion they phone back later if they have any further questions. One of the scenarios we ask our students to do is to tell an owner their kitten died under anaesthesia for routine neutering. Clearly, this can raise a lot of emotions in the client. But what this particular client is concerned about is how to tell his young daughter for whom the kitten was bought. This scenario resolves best when the student recognizes and acknowledges how difficult this situation is for the owner, and then provides a practical solution by offering to speak to their daughter with them. Empathy requires us to acknowledge our client's predicament, to show them that we understand and to provide practical solutions where possible.

Involving the client

The old way to practise medicine essentially centred on the health care professional. They knew best. Patients simply answered what they were asked, listened to what they were told, and followed instructions. There is now clear evidence that satisfaction and clinical outcome improve when the consultation revolves around the client and patient rather than around the health care professional (Abood 2007). We must aim to involve our clients in the decision-making process, and show that they themselves, their animals and their concerns are central to the consultation at all times.

Involving the animal

There is not an owner on the planet who does not appreciate it when a vet acknowledges their animals appropriately. There is almost always something positive and truthful that can be said. We should ignore the client's animal at our peril. I guess, as workers in the animal health industry, we tend to be quite good at this.

THE PHYSICAL EXAMINATION

In the model, the physical examination is sandwiched between gathering and giving information. Clearly, as we become more efficient, then we will start to merge these two processes. But we must never let the physical examination interfere with our communication. Clients may feel they are not being listened to if we are also examining a leg. We just need to explain to them what is happening. However, we should leave some time in the consultation for just communicating with our client. It is part of making them feel special and important, and will really help build up a good working relationship with them.

CLOSING THE CONSULTATION

The end of another consultation has arrived. Now is the time to make sure we are all singing from the same song sheet. We can achieve this through careful summarizing. At this stage we, as the professional, as well as our clients, need to be sure of our ongoing responsibilities. This includes what to do if the agreed plan is not working, and when and how our client should seek help. Just before we finish, we should check again that the client is happy with the outcome and ask if everything has been covered. 'Have I missed anything?' is my favourite question. I know this may raise some concerns about clients saying, 'Oh yes, whilst I am here, I did notice that . . .'. But if we established all the owner's concerns at the beginning of the consult, this is very unlikely. And it can be very satisfying when they say, 'No, thank you, that is everything'. Finally, it only remains to thank the client and say goodbye . . . and then it all starts again with the next one.

SUMMARY

Some people raise concerns that applying such a model as this will lead to impossibly long consultations. However, the evidence from our medical colleagues is that good communication developed within such frameworks is more efficient and does not take any extra time (Marvel et al. 1998). Other people are concerned that following such an apparently strict methodology will remove their individuality as communicators. However, that really is not what this is about. There is endless scope within the model to develop our own style, and it is very important we do. We are not actors, and we cannot deliver a script. We can, however, talk from the heart. And if we use a model like this one, we can break the consultation down into manageable chunks, allowing us to evaluate our own consultation style in a logical framework, and improve our own performance. The evidence is clear – we can all learn to consult better. And if we do, we will enjoy our jobs more, have more satisfied clients, and last, but not least, have healthier patients.

REFERENCES

Abood SK (2007) Increasing adherence in practice: making your clients partners in care. *Veterinary Clinics of North America: Small Animal Practice* 37(1):151–164.

Beckman HB, Frankel RM (1984) The effect of physician behavior on the collection of data. *Annals of Internal Medicine* 101(5):692–696.

Haslam N (2007) Humanising medical practice: the role of empathy. *Medical Journal of Australia* 187(7):381–382.

Marvel MK, Doherty WJ, Weiner E (1998) Medical interviewing by exemplary family physicians. *Journal of Family Practice* 47(5):343–348.

Radford A, Stockley P, Silverman J, Taylor I, Turner R, Gray C, Bush L, Glyde M, Healy A, Dale V, Kaney S, Magrath C, Marshall S, May S, McVey B, Spencer C, Sutton R, Tandy R, Watson P, Winter A (2006) Development, teaching, and evaluation of a consultation structure model for use in veterinary education. *Journal of Veterinary Medical Education* 33(1):38–44.

Silverman J, Kurtz S, Draper J (2006) *Skills for Communicating with Patients*, 2nd edn. Radcliffe Medical, Abingdon, UK.

Stepien KA, Baernstein A (2006) Educating for empathy: a review. *Journal of General Internal Medicine* 21:524–530.

Professional, ethical and legal aspects of communication

Carol Gray

Introduction

The legal basis of the veterinary surgeon–client relationship is contract. The contract in this case is between the client, who either brings an animal to the veterinary practice or requests a visit to home or business premises, and the professional whom they have consulted for veterinary services. Professional behaviour and an appropriate attitude to this contract are therefore important components of veterinary surgeon–client communications. In the first half of the consultation, the process of gathering information from clients is governed by professional ethical (confidentiality) and legal (data protection legislation) boundaries. However, it is the second half of the consultation, giving information to clients, that involves the more contentious and ethically challenging debates surrounding informed decision making and consent. This chapter looks at some of the communication issues involved in these areas.

COMMUNICATING PROFESSIONALISM

Many aspects of our personality are conveyed in our communication style, including non-verbal and verbal behaviours. It is essential that members of a professional practice team convey a suitable attitude via how they appear, what they say and what they do. A major part of this projection is to get the 'preparation' phase of communication right. Preparation allows you to check your appearance and the environment, to get rid of any baggage from previous consultations or encounters, and to greet the client with a professional state of mind.

The definition of professional appearance may vary between practices and clients. Research carried out in medicine has produced variable results. In one survey, patients preferred doctors to wear a white coat rather than scrubs, business dress or casual dress and felt

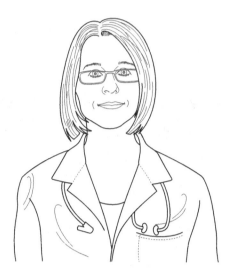

Figure 3.1 Professional appearance instills trust and confidence.

that such attire instilled trust and confidence (Rehman et al. 2005). This confirms the findings of an earlier survey, which showed that 49% of patients in an emergency department thought that doctors should wear a white coat (Colt & Solot 1989). However, a survey of outpatients in an obstetrics and gynaecology department showed that they had no preference between doctors in business attire, casual clothing or scrub suits (Figure 3.1) (Fischer et al. 2007).

A larger range of options were given to patients in a New Zealand study, with semi-formal (blouse or shirt/tie with dark coloured skirt or trousers) attire being the preferred option, over formal attire with white coat. The addition of a smile improved the score for all styles of clothing. Items of clothing or appearance that were disliked by patients included facial piercings, brightly dyed hair, long hair in men, long earrings, short tops or skirts in women, T-shirts, training shoes and sandals. Interestingly, a tie depicting a cartoon character was more disliked than no tie at all (Lill & Wilkinson 2005). Although these studies refer to patients' impressions of their doctors' appearance, it would be reasonable to generalize the findings to any medical setting, including veterinary practices. A professional appearance is important in getting the veterinarian–client relationship off to a good start. However, it appears that this aspect of professionalism is not as important to patients as other attributes such as compassion and having plenty of time for them (Wiggins et al. 2009).

Methods of opening the consultation or interview will vary too, with everyone having an individual style. What does the literature suggest as best practice for a professional greeting? In a telephone survey of 415 patients, 78.1% wanted their doctor to shake hands with them at the start of the consultation, but, interestingly, older patients were less likely to want their doctor to shake hands (Makoul et al. 2007). Although shaking hands when greeting others is less common among people in general today, it still seems to convey a message of professionalism.

Name badges and formal introductions also seem to be important in radiating a professional manner. In one survey, 76% of patients thought that a doctor should always wear a name badge, with most preferring the breast pocket as the ideal site (Lill & Wilkinson 2005).

In the same survey, the preferred method of introduction by the doctor was title, first and second name, for example, 'My name is Dr John Smith'. Whatever the practice protocol on dress and introductions, the client's preference for how they wish to be addressed should be elicited ('What would you like me to call you?' or 'Is it all right to call you Mr Bradley?').

GATHERING INFORMATION FROM CLIENTS

Data protection and client confidentiality

Information is gathered from clients as soon as they enter the veterinary practice, starting in the waiting room. Is there any legal aspect to this information gathering? In the UK, the Data Protection Act 1984 sets out obligations regarding storage and use of personal details, and the rights of individuals to request access to their records. It is therefore important to bear this in mind when writing clinical records. Clinical records must be accurate, up-to-date and free from any insulting language or abbreviations/acronyms, as clients are entitled to have these explained to them. As the Royal College of Veterinary Surgeons (RCVS) Guide to Professional Conduct (2008a) states:

> It follows that the utmost care is essential in writing case notes or recording a client's personal details to ensure that the latter are accurate (particularly in relation to financial details) and that the notes are comprehensible and legible.

There are also problems over ownership of radiographs and other images. The RCVS suggests that fees could be 'for diagnosis or advice only' rather than for taking radiographs. If clients are specifically charged for radiographs, they are entitled to have them (RCVS 2008a).

The Data Protection Act also governs closed-circuit television images. They must be stored securely, and only for as long as necessary. However, video recording for research/training purposes requires specific consent from the client. This is discussed later.

As stated in the opening paragraph, the legal basis of the transaction between the animal owner and the veterinary practice is contract. The contract is for the practice to provide a service to the client. Some practices have written contracts for clients to agree to before they will provide a service (known as 'terms of business'). Usual contract rules apply. The three components of a contract are offer, acceptance and consideration. There must be an offer from the practice to provide the service (it does not need to be in writing). The offer becomes legally binding once the client has accepted it (the acceptance). Again, this does not need to be in writing. The consideration is the price the client pays for the service. From a legal aspect, there must be the intention to create legal relations, but all commercial agreements are assumed to have this basis. The offer is made as an advertised (fixed) or estimated cost of treatment, often written into the consent process. By signing the form, or verbally agreeing to treatment in the consulting room or on the farm, the client is accepting the offer, and becomes legally bound to pay the consideration if the service is performed. We return to contract and consent later in this chapter.

One interesting aspect of communication with clients is the notion of 'client confidentiality', a principle that has been upheld as an essential component of professional conduct. However, this is being gradually eroded as more exceptions to the maintenance of confidentiality are listed. For example, confidentiality can be broken in suspected cases of animal abuse or disputes over ownership of a microchipped animal (note that in the UK, the RCVS should be consulted first). Client records may be requested in court proceedings or at RCVS disciplinary hearings.

If a client has come from another practice, it is ethical (and polite) to contact the previous practice. What if the client refuses to agree to this? It can be written into practice policy that only those new clients who allow contact with, and access to records from, previous veterinary practices, will be taken on. It is more appropriate to cite animal welfare as the main reason for this (for example, prevention of repeating tests already carried out), rather than professional courtesy.

Client confidentiality is also broken in cases of referrals (implied consent can be assumed if the client requests the referral, but consent to pass on details should be obtained if the veterinary surgeon suggests this course of action) and for insurance claims (although, again, implied consent is assumed if the client brings in the claim form for completion). We look at implied consent later in this chapter.

In the USA, the issue of veterinarian–client confidentiality is even more confusing. In some states (e.g. Kansas), there are statutory confidentiality requirements in veterinary practice acts. In others (e.g. Louisiana), state veterinary medical boards have broad confidentiality regulations, which although less 'weighty' than state legislation, can lead to disciplinary action if they are breached (Babcock & Pfeiffer 2006).

GIVING INFORMATION TO CLIENTS

Informed decision making

The minefield of giving information to clients can be made slightly more negotiable by remembering the reasons for giving the information. Traditionally, there was an overwhelming air of paternalism about the veterinary consultation, with veterinary surgeons held in high esteem and revered for their knowledge about animal disease and treatment, which they did not choose to share with their clients.

The aim in most modern-day veterinary practices, especially companion animal practices, is to involve the client in shared decision making that takes into account the unique human–animal bond (Figure 3.2) and the client's individual circumstances. In order to enable the client to make an informed decision, the veterinary surgeon, as the partner with professional knowledge, skills and experience, should aim to provide the client with all of the information necessary to make the decision. This, in itself, can cause problems.

First, the options for treatment need to be presented to the client in accessible language. How much does the client know already? It is vitally important to find out the client's starting point and to tailor the explanations accordingly. This is an area of veterinary communication that appears to require some practice. In a small pilot study carried out at the University of Liverpool, in none of the recorded consultations did the veterinary surgeon find out about the client's level of knowledge and experience (Gray et al. 2005).

Many veterinary surgeons will present only one or two options for treatment, leaving out other options totally for a variety of reasons. These reasons may be client-based (perceived lack of money, doubts about client's ability to follow treatment instructions, incorrect assessment of human–animal bond) or veterinary surgeon-based (lack of experience of treatment

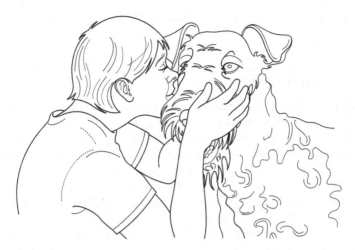

Figure 3.2 The human–animal bond.

option, desire to try out a new technique, reluctance to offer referral). This brings in ethical considerations. Is it ever ethical to withhold information from clients? A similar debate has recently taken place in medicine, where an article in the *British Medical Journal* on deceiving patients provoked a highly charged response (Sokol 2007).

When financial considerations are involved, the debate becomes very difficult for physicians. A survey of 1000 Californian doctors found that 46% of respondents disagreed with the statement: 'If a medical intervention has any chance (no matter how small) of helping the patient, it is the physician's duty to offer it regardless of cost' (Ginsburg et al. 2000).

So, what is good practice in giving information for shared decision making with clients? Some authors have proposed three basic communication styles: guardian, where the veterinarian provides the information and makes the decision; teacher, where the veterinarian provides information but the client also obtains information from other sources, and is responsible for making the decision; and collaborator, where the veterinarian and the client both provide information and reach a shared decision (Cornell & Kopcha 2007).

Initially, all the options should be listed, without further explanation (signposting – 'First I will tell you all of the options we have for treatment, including estimated costs'). This may include the 'do nothing' option, because it is often useful to explain what will happen if we do nothing. The client then realizes that a decision has to be made on the other options.

What about clients who do not wish to be involved in the decision-making process? There will always be a proportion of clients who want the veterinary surgeon to make the decision for them. A survey of human patients found that 52% wanted to leave decisions to their doctors, although interestingly, 96% of the same sample wanted to be offered choices and asked for their opinions (Levinson et al. 2005). In truly client- or relationship-centred practice, clients should be allowed their wishes to abdicate decision-making responsibilities. How can we make this safe for all concerned? In order to avoid problems with a decision taken solely by the veterinary surgeon, it is good practice to describe fully all the treatment options available, and then to explain why the particular option is chosen. It should be documented that this has been done on the clinical record, and the fact that the client requested that the veterinary surgeon makes the decision on treatment should also be documented.

Models of decision making

Two main models of decision making have been proposed. These are known as the 'agency-based' and the 'informed treatment' decision-making approaches (Gafni et al. 1998).

Each of these models gives a different role to the health care professional, but both acknowledge this role as being the professional one in the relationship. As Gafni indicates, the choice of model requires a completely different approach by the veterinary surgeon. If the client wishes the veterinary surgeon to make the decision, it is important that the role adopted is that of a 'perfect agent' (Evans 1984), both for the client and for the patient. This means that the veterinary surgeon must endeavour to discover the client's preferences, where the animal fits into their life, and must act as an advocate for the animal regarding the best choice for quality of life/welfare.

To take on the role of perfect agent, the veterinary surgeon must work hard during the first half of the consultation, gathering information from the client about, for example, their hopes, concerns, financial situation and expectations, while carefully observing and examining the patient and evaluating the human–animal bond. The decision on preferred treatment is made by the veterinary surgeon, but based on the information gathered from the client and from examination of the patient. As mentioned above, the options, plus costs and benefits of each, should still be carefully explained to the client and documented as such.

The second model, informed decision making by the client, requires the veterinary surgeon to act as the source of technical and professional knowledge, which is shared with the client in such a way as to enable them to make a decision.

With this option, the client's preferences, motivation, financial situation, etc., may not even become apparent (although it is still good practice to find out the client's ideas, concerns and expectations during the first half of the consultation; see Chapter 2).

This model of decision making requires exemplary communication skills from the veterinary surgeon. Clients must be given the information about the treatment options in language free from jargon, in bite-sized chunks with opportunities for clarification and questions, with frequent summarizing to aid recall and without bias towards one option over another (unless there is a clear welfare concern with any of the options).

Decision making in practice

As an example, we will consider the decision-making process for a dog with a severely traumatized right forelimb following a road accident. There is a compound, comminuted fracture of the radius and ulna, with extensive degloving injury from elbow to carpus. Assuming that the dog has been given appropriate first-aid treatment, we now have to guide the owner through the decision-making process.

We can first of all explain why doing nothing is not an option (compromised welfare via infection, non-union, pain). We are left with three options: attempt to salvage the limb in this practice, refer for salvage surgery and amputate the limb. How should we present the options?

First, we should signpost the three options:

> Mr Client, there are three options for treating these injuries – we can try to save the leg in this practice, we can refer Dog for treatment at a local referral hospital or we can decide to amputate the leg.

The client already knows the extent and severity of the injuries, so the mention of amputation should not be too much of a shock to him. We can then go on to explain in more detail the costs (not just financial) and benefits of each option. A suggested checklist of factors to consider in this case is as follows:

- Non-treatable injuries
- Available expertise
- Financial constraints
- Concurrent injuries
- Patient factors
- Owners' commitment
- Welfare implications
- Cost–benefit analysis (Ness 2002)

The patient should have been assessed for non-treatable and concurrent injuries at the initial presentation. Any damage to nerve or blood supply would rule out a salvage operation, but the owner should still be told why this option is impossible. The expertise of available staff should not influence the decision whether to salvage or amputate – if there is no one capable of performing the surgery in the practice, then referral would be the method of salvage.

We will assume that there is an experienced orthopaedic surgeon available in the practice, but there is also a referral hospital 10 miles away with an orthopaedic specialist and an intensive care unit.

In presenting our three treatment options, we would therefore take a non-judgemental approach:

> So, Mr Client, let's go through the three options carefully. In my opinion, the leg is salvageable, but it will be a long and intensive healing process. Mr Bone is our orthopaedic surgeon in the practice, and he can perform the surgery to try to get the pieces of bone back together and to get the skin wound to heal. It will involve many repeated visits to the surgery and several surgical procedures for Dog. We are talking about an expensive series of operations, bandages, X-rays, etc. I'd estimate we are talking around £x000 in total. It will require an ongoing commitment from you to keep an eye on things at home, to keep bringing Dog regularly for check-ups and bandage changes, probably under sedation or general anaesthesia, so you might have to leave him for several hours. However, I think the chances of eventually having a useful leg are good. Have I explained that well enough? Do you have any questions about this option at the moment?

After each treatment option, it is good practice to check on the client's understanding, and invite any questions, before proceeding to the next option.

> We also have the option of sending Dog to Topdog Hospital for treatment. It will be more expensive, but they have the latest equipment and are trained in the latest techniques for this type of surgery. They could possibly give Dog a higher chance of a very good result. They will be more expensive, and it is further to travel for you and for Dog, especially if you need to leave him for treatment. Your commitment to the treatment will therefore be higher. I'm afraid I cannot give you an estimated cost, but I can find out a figure for you before you make your decision. Do you have any other questions about this option?

Again, after presenting the pros and cons for this option, the client is given the opportunity to ask for clarification or for any additional information.

> Finally, we can consider amputation. Although this will give the poorest result cosmetically, it will return Dog to being pain-free in the shortest time. He is small enough to be able to get around pretty well on three legs and, as far as we know, dogs don't have psychological problems with losing a leg. It is also the least expensive and most quantifiable treatment financially, as it is a single procedure. We would charge approximately £x00 for this; that's an estimate as we can't predict how long the surgery will take. Is that information enough for you to make a decision? Is there anything else we need to discuss?

The next factor to consider is the length of time the client can take to decide. Obviously, the dog cannot be left for too long before further treatment is carried out. However, the client needs to go through the options, and will possibly need to discuss them with other members of the family. There may be financial enquiries to carry out (some owners will even re-mortgage houses or take out personal loans to pay for veterinary treatment).

Notice that we have not mentioned insurance yet. This is deliberate. We should not allow insurance to influence decision making. All options should be presented before enquiring whether the animal is insured. We should never rule out an option in an uninsured animal on grounds of expense. We cannot possibly know the client's financial situation, or how far the client is willing to go to find the money. A survey of doctors in the USA found that clinical decisions in non-life-threatening cases varied depending on the patients' type of insurance, and the influence of this factor on decision making was stressful for the doctors involved (Shen et al. 2004).

We have presented the three options with advantages and disadvantages of each. Are there any other ways we can help the client to decide?

We can also look at the quality of life. This is an area of veterinary science that is receiving increased interest and attention (Anon 2006). With chronic conditions, there can be a problem with assessing how the animal is responding to the treatment. If we can help clients to assess and monitor quality of life in the animals they live with, this can be a useful tool to help with decision making. How can we do this? Recently, a quality-of-life questionnaire has been designed and evaluated for owners to use (Wojciechowska et al. 2005). This assesses non-physical quality of life, and could be used with a patient who is suffering from a chronic disease, to help the owner to decide whether the treatment is working, and whether to go on. Indeed, Rollin (2006) suggests that an essential part of the veterinarian–client relationship should be to ask the client, who knows the animal better than anyone, to be involved in helping to define quality of life for that animal, at an early stage. Veterinary surgeons can then keep the quality of life for the animal as the central focus in decision making, and this can make end-of-life decisions, in particular, more of a joint venture rather than a decision taken by the veterinary surgeon. Again, there will be clients who will not want to be involved in making the decision, and this should be respected. See Chapter 4 for more information on decision making and euthanasia.

Decision making often leads to the necessity to obtain consent from the client for the proposed treatment option.

INFORMED CONSENT

'Informed consent' is an emerging area of concern in veterinary practice. It is probably accurate to suggest that we are light years behind medicine in our approach to the topic (although the practical experiences of the consent process in medicine are sometimes far removed from the theoretical aspects discussed in the relevant literature).

So, what is 'informed consent'? According to Flemming and Scott (2004), the consent process for veterinary procedures should contain the following:

- The diagnosis or nature of the patient's ailment
- The general nature of the proposed treatment and any alternative
- Treatments and the purpose or reason for each treatment
- The risks or dangers involved in the proposed treatments
- The probability or prospects of success with each alternative treatment
- The prognosis or risk if the client refuses treatment
- The costs of the various alternative treatments
- If the treatment involves surgery, the individual who will actually perform that surgery if not the same as the individual obtaining consent
- The location and method of transportation to that location if the treatment is to be administered at another site

Can we draw parallels between consent in medicine and veterinary medicine? At first glance, the answer would seem to be 'no'. Consent in human medicine was famously defined by the presiding judge in a case in the USA, where a surgeon failed to obtain consent for a hysterectomy:

Every human being of adult years and sound mind has a right to determine what shall be done with his own body. (Schloendorff vs Society of New York Hospital 1914)

Surgery without consent in humans is described in criminal terms as 'battery' (Aitkenhead 2006). Does the same offence apply to surgery without consent in animals? Well, the answer is no, and further investigation reveals why not.

It concerns the legal status of animals. Although there have been moves to change this, especially in the USA, animals are still regarded as their owners' property, to do with as they wish, subject to animal welfare and animal health legislation.

There has been a campaign in the USA to have animals recognized as 'sentient property' (Matlack 2004) and owners reclassified as 'guardians', both of which would have a substantial impact on animal law.

Currently, consent for surgery on an animal involves the owner's consent as a 'surrogate' or 'proxy'. Any unlawful surgery on the animal creates an offence of 'trespass', or interference with someone's property without consent. However, the dissimilarities do not end there. Medical consent involves a mainly ethical process: '. . . respect for autonomy and self-determination of patients' (Bernat 2002), whereas consent for veterinary procedures also involves a contract between the client and the veterinary practice, and this can complicate matters. Most consent forms also constitute written contracts, involving estimates (or, less frequently, quotes) for the treatment involved (see Chapter 5). This can take the emphasis away from the actual consent procedure. Indeed, some sources recommend a move towards having separate forms for recording the consent process and the financial contract (Dye 2006).

The blurred distinction between consent and contract also appears when considering who can legally give consent. In the UK, persons of 16 years and more can give medical consent for procedures (General Medical Council 1998). However, in England a contract is only valid if both parties are 18 years or more (Family Law Reform Act 1969). In Scotland, the age limit for contract is 16.

Many practices are unsure of where to set the age limit for consent but, in view of the necessity to collect adequate fees for veterinary services, 18 years of age would seem to be a sensible age limit. This also brings us to the question of who can obtain consent. It certainly suggests that a 17-year-old veterinary nurse is an unsuitable person to do so.

What is the RCVS' advice on consent and fees?

> When dealing directly with the owner, or the owner's agent whose consent to treatment must be given, it is important to obtain that consent in writing on a properly drafted form which should include any estimated charge. (RCVS 2008a)

The question of 'owner's agent' is an interesting one. What constitutes an 'owner's agent'? And what is their status in law? Certain agents are fairly obvious, for example, a racehorse trainer or greyhound trainer has a legal relationship with the owner. Similarly, a livery stable or boarding kennel owner would have an 'agency' clause written into a contract with the owner. The situation becomes tricky when dealing with non-formalized relationships. Family members can act as agents in the absence of the owner, but there have been cases of malicious agency, for example, the estranged husband or wife requesting euthanasia of the partner's animal. To be absolutely safe, all owners' agents should have written 'authority to act' signed by the owner. However, any veterinary surgeon who takes reasonable steps to confirm ownership of an animal cannot be held responsible in cases of malicious misrepresentation.

This may be as simple as asking of anyone bringing in an animal for treatment 'Who is the owner?' and documenting the reply in the clinical records.

What constitutes informed consent? In reality, 'informed consent' does not exist as a legal term. It is accepted that for any consent to be valid in law, it must be informed. In practice, we can divide the term up into its component parts – firstly, informing the patient (client) and, secondly, documenting the process (Childers et al. 2009).

In the UK, the RCVS advises that veterinary surgeons should:

> obtain the client's informed consent to treatment unless delay would adversely affect the animal's welfare (to give informed consent, clients must be aware of risks)

and, expanding on this advice,

> informed consent can only be given by a client who has had the opportunity to consider the options for treatment, and had the significance and risks explained to them. (RCVS 2008a)

Compare this with the advice on consent available to medical colleagues. Valid consent to medical treatment is made up of three main components:

1. Adequate information for the patient to make a rational decision
2. Capacity (competence) of the patient to make a decision
3. Decision freely made without coercion (Bernat 2002)

However, the RCVS has produced additional notes on consent and contract in response to the high numbers of complaints involving consent issues (RCVS 2008b).

Communication of risk

The information given to the patient (in the medical environment) should include options for treatment and 'material risks' of each. A material risk is one to which a reasonable person in the patient's position would attach significance (Aitkenhead 2006). For example, with a general anaesthetic, the risk of death, although small, is a material risk. There is some debate over whether postoperative complications should be included, but this is particularly relevant to human patients as they may not regain consciousness and be able to make the decision in that situation. With animals, the owner could be contacted for consent in a similar situation.

There is a wealth of research in medicine on how best to communicate risk and the size of that risk. This has valid application to veterinary medicine. In order to make an informed decision, clients must be made aware of the risks involved with a proposed treatment or surgical procedure. Under UK law, the legal standards for disclosure of risk in medicine are 'what a reasonable doctor would disclose' (Palmboom et al. 2007). In the same paper, it was discovered that the most difficult situation for clinicians to decide whether to disclose is in the 'very low risk – very severe complication' end of the probability–severity spectrum. This may include the risk of death in general anaesthesia of healthy animals, but it would seem sensible that this risk falls into the 'material risk' category.

According to Epstein et al. (2004), the clinician should differentiate evidence-based recommendations from those generated by personal experience or bias, including financial or convenience factors. However, in the era of clinical audit, it is suggested that individual practice records relating to success of treatments or risks of general anaesthesia should be equally valid.

The way in which risks are presented to the client may have a bearing on the resulting decision. Risk framing refers to the way in which the absolute risk is described. For example, 'this will affect one in 100 animals' is viewed differently to '99 out of 100 animals will not be affected' (Crowson et al. 2006). The suggested solution is to use both phrases simultaneously: 'out of 100 animals, one will be affected and 99 will not'.

Interestingly, although studies have shown that people understand graphical displays of risk (bar charts, pie graphs or icons) more easily than numerical presentations (Edwards et al. 2002), there is also evidence that they find numerical risk information less threatening (Timmermans et al. 2004).

Klein and Stefanek (2007) looked at patients' understanding of numerical information and found that they tended to overestimate risk and place too much weight on the numerators (top line) of fractions. Their suggestion was to present risk as a percentage (e.g. 8%) along with two or more frequencies and associated denominators (e.g. 8 of 100 or 80 of 1000). The advice to prevent risk framing described above should also be used with these presentations.

Why does this matter? A review by Trevana et al. (2006) found that clinician training in a patient-centred approach to risk communication led to improved patient satisfaction, knowledge, perception and consultation processes.

Competence to give consent

With animals, the second criterion of informed consent is never achievable, as we are always dealing with 'never-competent' patients. This puts animals on the same level as infants and preschool children, incapable of making decisions or expressing their wishes.

Surrogate or proxy consent, which always applies to consent given by veterinary clients, consists of three levels of decision making. The preferred level is 'expressed wishes', where the patient has indicated what they would like to happen by writing it down (e.g. living wills). The next level is 'substituted judgement', where the proxy bases the decision on the patient's values and treatment preferences as understood by them. With animals, the third level is the only method possible, where the patient's 'best interests' are calculated by looking at benefits of treatment and burdens to the patient (Bernat & Peterson 2006).

The professional expertise of the veterinary surgeon allows the owner to make this type of decision, by providing all the necessary information. It is not the veterinary surgeon's responsibility to make the decision, unless the owner is not contactable and it is an emergency situation.

Bernat and Peterson (2006) describe the process of consent as 'an ongoing bidirectional process of communication, education, question answering and listening'. How do we achieve this ideal in veterinary practice?

The 'two-way' communication described comprises two essential components – giving the information (adequate explanation of the procedures and their alternatives, and the risks involved with each) and an indication of understanding (comprehension of these procedures and risks). How does this work in practice? As discussed in Chapter 2 and earlier in this chapter, giving information to clients involves well-defined communication skills, including the giving of small pieces of information and checking for understanding of each ('chunking and checking'), avoiding the use of jargon and structuring the information by the use of signposting and summarizing. This also applies to the consent process. Here is an example, involving a suspected gastric foreign body.

> In summary, Ms Client, we have discussed the reasons for your visit today, and we have decided that Puppy needs further investigation for his vomiting. We have several options. We could wait and see, we could do some diagnostic X-rays, and, in both cases, we could end up having to do an operation. I'll take you through these one at a time.

Here, the veterinary surgeon is using signposting to structure the explanation for the client.

> First of all, if we wait and see, by giving some anti-vomiting treatment, and observing Puppy for the rest of the day, we avoid having to give Puppy an anaesthetic. Unfortunately, I feel that Puppy may have eaten something, and if I am right, he will get worse during the day and be in a worse condition if we have to anaesthetize him later. Does that make sense to you?

The veterinary surgeon uses chunking and checking to present the options to the client.

> Our second option is to give Puppy a general anaesthetic to allow us to take some X-rays of his tummy. If he has eaten something, we should see it on the X-ray. We would then know what we are dealing with and what we have to do next. The drawback is that if we let him wake up, he may need another anaesthetic to carry out the surgery. Have I explained that clearly?

> Our third option is to give him a general anaesthetic with a view to taking the X-rays, but also going on to do any surgery required. This will mean a longer anaesthetic, but will avoid having to give a second anaesthetic. Have I explained that well enough?

The veterinary surgeon then summarizes the three options for the client and screens to check that the client has no further questions. It is suggested that it is good practice to keep screening, by asking, 'Do you have any further questions?' until the client says, 'No' (Flemming & Scott 2004).

> So, to sum up, we can do a bit of a 'wait and see', but Puppy's condition may get worse, we can give a short anaesthetic to take X-rays, or we can give a longer anaesthetic to take X-rays but also go on to do any surgery required, for instance, to remove any object we see on X-ray. Is that okay? Do you have any questions about the options?

Obviously, this extract merely introduces the options for treatment in this case, and does not include discussion of the risks of general anaesthesia or of the possible surgical procedure. The veterinary surgeon indicates the preferred option. Is this ethically correct?

The client has consulted the veterinary surgeon for a professional opinion. It is perfectly acceptable for the professional to indicate the medically preferred option; after all, the client does not have equivalent medical knowledge. However, bear in mind that consent must never be coerced from a client. One example of this is using the phrase, 'if it was my dog, I would . . .', which can be regarded as emotional blackmail. Veterinary surgeons can never put themselves in clients' shoes. It is better either to offer no opinion on which is the best option or to recommend an option using professional experience and medical knowledge without personal input (see earlier description of patterns of communication and decision-making models). However, this changes in cases of compromised animal welfare. If there is really only one option in terms of welfare, the veterinary surgeon has a responsibility to act as an advocate for the animal. After all, animal welfare comes above all else in the RCVS's ten guiding principles (RCVS 2008a).

A more extreme form of patient advocacy involves paying scant regard to the client's wishes, and advocating on behalf of the animal for the treatment that offers the best outcome with the least risk, regardless of costs (Fettman & Rollin 2002).

Refusal of consent for a procedure that is required to prevent pain and suffering to the animal can be a problem in veterinary practice, but the overwhelming duty of care is to the animal. In extreme cases, animal welfare organizations and/or the police may need to be involved. If the client is not present and an animal requires life-saving surgery, then the surgery can go ahead without consent. In fact, in this case, if the veterinary surgeon fails to carry out the surgery, or put an end to the animal's suffering in some way, it may well be considered an offence under the Animal Welfare Act 2006.

In the example above, all three of the treatment options may be equally valid. If the veterinary surgeon could not feel a foreign body on physical examination, then a 'wait-and-see' option is acceptable. If, however, a foreign body was palpable in the small intestines, and clinical signs showed that the puppy was unlikely to be able to pass it, then surgery is the only option and the client should be guided to this decision.

Now, what constitutes 'informed consent' in the above scenario? Let us assume that the client has opted for the second option, a general anaesthetic for abdominal X-rays, but has asked that the veterinary surgeon telephones her if the results suggest that surgery is required.

Here is the consent process:

Okay, Ms Client, we have decided to give Puppy a general anaesthetic to X-ray his abdomen, his tummy. Do you have any questions about what is going to happen?

Now, I'd like to go through the procedure with you. Puppy will be given a sedative, and then when he's quite sleepy, we will give him an injection of anaesthetic into his vein to send him to sleep. He will then have a tube placed into his windpipe and he will be given anaesthetic gas to keep him asleep. This will allow us to take pictures of his stomach. The X-ray procedure is quite safe, but the general anaesthetic has some risks associated with it. One of these risks, although it is extremely rare, is death. In our practice, the risk is less than 1 in 5000 animals. However, it is a risk, no matter how small. Another risk is vomiting while under anaesthetic, which can lead to choking or to pneumonia, if the vomit is inhaled. This is less of a risk once the tube is in place in Puppy's windpipe. Obviously, I have to advise you of these risks, although the chances of them happening to Puppy are small. I will be performing the procedure, assisted by a qualified veterinary nurse, who will monitor the anaesthetic. Do you have any questions about this information?

Please read the consent form. It details the conversation we have had. If anything is unclear, please ask me. If you are satisfied with the information, please sign it at the bottom.

Is there anything else that the veterinary surgeon could do to improve the consent process? It has been suggested that getting the client to repeat back the information ensures that they have understood (Lashley et al. 2000). This may be the 'gold standard' for informed consent, as it confirms that the client is (1) competent to make the decision, and (2) has been given the information in an appropriate format.

Should we mention death as a small, but significant, risk of anaesthesia? In order to obtain truly informed consent, then yes, we must. This is particularly important for veterinary surgery, as animals do have a higher risk of death than human patients under anaesthetic (see earlier section on communication of risk). Cats have a risk of death of 0.24% or 24 deaths per 10 000 (Brodbelt et al. 2007) compared to a human risk of 1.4 deaths per 10 000 (Arbous et al. 2001). Many veterinary surgeons feel uncomfortable mentioning the risk of death when obtaining consent for elective procedures on healthy animals, but it must be done or the consent is not valid. If the client then decides not to go ahead with the procedure, then that is their informed decision.

It is recommended that the risk of death should be clearly stated on the consent form for anaesthesia. For example, a form of words such as, 'I understand and accept that all treatments, anaesthesia and surgical techniques involve risk to the animal, including risk of death ...', would be suitable (Wright 1995).

A suggested pro forma for a consent form for anaesthesia and surgical procedures follows. In designing the 'ideal' consent form, the advice to have two separate forms has been heeded, and the need to mention the very low risk of a very severe complication (such as death) has been noted. Using the RCVS's own suggestion for a consent form (RCVS 2009) as a basis, the forms shown in Figures 3.3 and 3.4 are suggested as a model for consent for anaesthesia and surgical procedures in practice.

In the case described previously, the consent process is taking place immediately before the procedure will be carried out. This is the usual situation for emergency procedures. However, it is also common practice to obtain consent for elective procedures on the morning of the operation. Is this good practice?

In medicine, the current recommendation is that the consent process should take place in advance of admission for surgery/general anaesthesia. Goldblatt (2006) suggests that it is 'bad timing to present the consent form for the first time on the day of elective surgery, when all concerned have convened for one purpose'.

Some veterinary practices have a policy of seeing clients for appointments in advance of elective procedures, to go through the consent process with them. This often involves giving them a copy of the consent form to take home, so that any further questions can be dealt with when admitting the patient. This is good practice in obtaining consent, and ensures that the client has a copy of the form that they have signed.

Must consent be in writing? The answer is 'no', although it makes record keeping easier, and it is useful to give the client a copy of the form to take away. One instance where it may

PART 1 – FORM OF CONSENT FOR ANAESTHESIA AND SURGICAL PROCEDURES

Species and Breed _____

Name _____ Colour _____

Age _____   Sex   M _____ F _____ NM _____ NF_____

Microchip/Tattoo/Brand _____

Owner's Name _____

Address _____

_____

Home/Work* telephone_____Mobile _____
(*delete as appropriate)

Operation/Procedure _____

I hereby give permission for the administration of an anaesthetic to the above animal and to the surgical operation/procedure detailed on this form together with any procedures necessary to save life in an emergency. The nature of these procedures has been explained to me and I understand that all anaesthetic techniques and surgical procedures involve some risk to the animal, including the risk of death. I accept that the likely cost will be as detailed on the attached estimate, and that in the event of further treatment being required or of complications occurring which will give rise to additional costs, I shall be contacted as soon as practicable so that my consent to such additional costs may be obtained.

Notes and Instructions: _____

_____

_____

Signature _____

Owner/Agent Name (Block Capitals)_____

Address (if not owner) _____

_____

_____

Contact telephone no (if not owner) _____

Date of Signature _____

Figure 3.3 Suggested form of consent for anaesthesia and surgical procedures based on RCVS specimen form (with permission from the Royal College of Veterinary Surgeons).

PART 2 – CONTRACT FOR ANAESTHESIA/SURGICAL PROCEDURES (to be kept with part 1)

Name of animal _____

Nature of surgical procedure(s) _____

_____

The estimated cost of the procedures described above (tick as appropriate)

☐   will be: £_____

☐   will be within the range: £_____ to £_____

Inclusive of: VAT _____ Post-op Exam _____ Post-op Treatment ____

And I agree that I will pay for the treatment on collection of the animal

Signature _____

Date of signature _____

Figure 3.4 Suggested contract for anaesthesia and surgical procedures based on RCVS specimen form (with permission from the Royal College of Veterinary Surgeons).

be more humane to accept verbal rather than written consent is the terminal patient who has arrived for euthanasia with a distressed owner. The insistence on written consent may only increase the risk of responsibility grief (see Chapter 4) with this type of client. Indeed, the Association of Anaesthetists of Great Britain and Ireland do not believe that a formal signed consent form is necessary for anaesthesia, as a signed consent form does not increase the validity of consent (Aitkenhead 2006).

Consent for anaesthesia and consent for euthanasia are quite different, however. It is useful to compile a checklist on practice policy for different situations involving requests for euthanasia, which may look as follows:

1. *New client with new patient* – Check ownership carefully and obtain written consent.
2. *Known client with new patient* – Again, check ownership carefully (some people have been known to 'kidnap' local problem animals and request euthanasia – why have you not seen this animal before?). Obtain written consent.

3. *Known patient with new client* – It may be that this is a member of the family that you have yet met, but it is sensible to check ownership (or agency) carefully and obtain written consent.
4. *Known client and patient* – If you have been discussing the timing of euthanasia over several consultations, and the time has arrived, then verbal consent is kinder for everyone. You have plenty of written evidence that this has been carefully planned.
5. *Telephone consent, for example, if a patient is anaesthetized on the operating table* – It is recommended that, if possible, two people listen to the client's verbal consent and everything is carefully documented. Obviously, the other requirements for consent should be present, i.e. that the client is competent to make the decision and that they have had their choices clearly explained to them.

A suggested pro forma for a consent form for euthanasia is shown in Figure 3.5. This is a model of a form for written consent for euthanasia, again, based on the RCVS version (RCVS 2008c).

Implied consent

The concept of implied consent is interesting. If a person, by their actions, suggests that they are consenting to a procedure, then implied consent is valid. When in hospital, for example, the act of opening one's mouth to have a thermometer inserted is taken as implied consent to having one's temperature taken, and a consent form does not have to be signed for this (Dye 2006). We can use this premise to argue that a consent process is not required for animals presented to the veterinary surgeon for treatment or vaccination. The action of bringing the animal to the surgery, or requesting a visit by the veterinary surgeon, is surely enough to imply consent by the client? However, it may be implied, but is it informed? It could be argued that certain side effects or severe reactions to drugs or vaccinations are common enough to require explicit consent from clients. This need not be in writing, but it is good practice to document that the client was informed of these risks before the vaccination or drug was given. In the case of 'off-label' use, where the drug or vaccine being used is not licensed for use in that species (e.g. most drugs used for treatment of exotic animals), written and informed consent is advisable.

Consent for research

What about consent for research and for procedures that are perhaps not in the best interests of the animal? Research may involve the animal being used for a clinical trial or the client being involved in research into attitudinal aspects of owning animals.

Clinical trials involve the testing of a veterinary medicinal product after administration of the correct dosage (Directive 2001/82/EEC 2001). They can be either dose-confirmation studies or verification studies to test the acceptability and efficacy of the product (Dennison & Leach 2006). It is necessary to obtain the informed consent of the client before enrolling a patient in a clinical trial:

[T]he informed consent of the owner of the animals to be used in the trial shall be obtained and documented . . . (Directive 2001/82/EEC)

FORM OF CONSENT FOR EUTHANASIA

Species and Breed _____

Name _____

Colour _____

Age _____   Sex   M/ F/ NM/ NF

Microchip/Tattoo/Brand _____

Owner's Name _____

Address _____

_____

Telephone: Home _____

               Work _____

               Mobile _____

I hereby confirm that:

☐   I am the owner of the animal described above OR

☐   I have the authority of the owner of the animal described above

And I request euthanasia of the animal

Signature _____

Name (Block Capitals) _____

Address (if not owner) _____

_____

_____

Contact Telephone No (if not owner) _____

Date of Signature _____

Figure 3.5   Suggested form of consent for euthanasia based on RCVS specimen form (with permission from the Royal College of Veterinary Surgeons).

Informed consent for clinical trials must be non-coercive, and include the reassurance that participation is voluntary, with no effect on subsequent veterinary treatment by the practice, should the client refuse. The client must be given full details of the drug or product being tested, possible risks or side effects and whom to contact should there be a problem. Practice staff should also be aware of which clients and patients are participating in the study, in case of adverse reactions.

While, in the above situation, consent must be obtained from clients on behalf of their animals, there may be some research carried out in practice that involves clients themselves. Research on human subjects involves the four principles outlined by Beauchamp and Childress (1994).

The principle of *justice* includes the right to privacy (e.g. anonymization of results) and the right to fair treatment (whether choosing to participate or not). The principle of *autonomy* involves being given all the information needed to make an informed decision without coercion. It is good practice to give all potential participants a written information sheet containing the following details:

- The purpose of the study
- Why they have been chosen
- That participation is optional and will not affect their treatment
- Description of what will happen should they participate
- Disadvantages of participation
- Benefits of participation
- Complaints
- Confidentiality
- What will happen to results
- Who is funding the research
- Ethical review
- Contact details for the researcher and practice staff involved (Pullen 2006)

The principle of *non-maleficence* requires that the researcher avoids doing harm to the participant. This may involve sourcing qualified counsellors who can provide appropriate support for the participants if required.

The principle of *beneficence* means that the researcher should try to maximize the good for the participant. The participant may get a feeling of satisfaction through taking part, feeling that they have benefited others by doing so, but it also helps to share the results with participants should they wish.

Consent for video-recording consultations for any purpose (research, postgraduate training, etc.) involves the same consent process with clients. It is good practice to obtain consent before the consultation, but also to give clients the option of changing their minds after the consultation. This can be achieved by asking them to sign an agreement that they are still happy to have the video included after the consultation has ended.

Consent for donation by animals is an important subsection of consent, where there is no obvious benefit to the patient. The client may feel a sense of satisfaction in that they have used their own animal to help another animal, but there can only be risks, and no benefits, for the donor animal. It is therefore up to each individual client to decide on a personal ethical viewpoint for this situation, and no client should be coerced into agreeing to allow an animal to donate blood or other tissue.

REFERENCES

Aitkenhead AR (2006) Informing and consenting for anaesthesia. *Best Practice and Research in Clinical Anaesthesiology* 20(4):507–524.

Anon (2006) What do we mean by quality of life? *Veterinary Record* 159:430–431.

Arbous MS, Grobbee DE, van Kleef JW, de Lange JJ, Spoormans HHAJM, Touw P, Werner FM, Meursing AEE (2001) Mortality associated with anaesthesia: a qualitative analysis to identify risk factors. *Anaesthesia* 56(12):1141–1153.

Babcock SL, Pfeiffer C (2006) Laws and regulations concerning the confidentiality of veterinarian-client communication. *Journal of the American Veterinary Medical Association* 229(3):365–369.

Beauchamp TL, Childress JE (1994) *Principles of Biomedical Ethics*. Oxford University Press, Oxford.

Bernat JL (2002) Informed consent in pediatric neurology. *Seminars in Pediatric Neurology* 9(1):10–18.

Bernat JL, Peterson LM (2006) Patient-centered informed consent in surgical practice. *Archives of Surgery* 141: 86–92.

Brodbelt DC, Pfeiffer DU, Young LE, Wood JL (2007) Risk factors for anaesthetic-related deaths in cats: results from the confidential enquiry into perioperative small animal fatalities. *British Journal of Anaesthesiology* 99:617–623.

Childers R, Lipsett PA, Pawlik TM (2009) Informed consent and the surgeon. *Journal of the American College of Surgeons* 208(4):627–634.

Colt HG, Solot JA (1989) Attitudes of patients and physicians regarding physician dress and demeanor in the emergency department. *Annals of Emergency Medicine* 18(2):145–151.

Cornell KK, Kopcha M (2007) Client-veterinarian communication: skills for client centered dialogue and shared decision-making. *Veterinary Clinics of North America: Small Animal* 37:37–47.

Crowson CS, Therneau T, Matteson EL, Gabriel SE (2006) Primer: demystifying risk – understanding and communicating medical risk. *Nature Clinical Practice in Rheumatology* 3:181–187.

Dennison T, Leach M (2006) Animal research, ethics and law. In: Pullen S, Gray C (eds), *Ethics, Law and the Veterinary Nurse*. Elsevier, Edinburgh.

Directive 2001/82/EC (2001) Official Journal of the European Communities.

Dye K (2006) Consent to treatment in veterinary practice. In: Pullen S, Gray C (eds), *Ethics, Law and the Veterinary Nurse*. Elsevier, Edinburgh.

Edwards A, Elwyn G, Mulley A (2002) Explaining risks: turning numerical data in to meaningful pictures. *British Medical Journal* 324:827–830.

Epstein RM, Alper BS, Quill TE (2004) Communicating evidence for participatory decision making. *JAMA* 291(19):2359–2366.

Evans RG (1984) *Strained Mercy: The Economics of Canadian Health Care*. Butterworths, Toronto, Canada.

Family Law Reform Act (1969) HMSO, London.

Fettman MJ, Rollin BE (2002) Modern elements of informed consent for general veterinary practitioners. *Journal of the American Veterinary Medical Association* 221(10):1386–1393.

Fischer RL, Hansen CE, Hunter RL, Veloski JJ (2007) Does physician attire influence patient satisfaction in an outpatient obstetrics and gynecology setting? *American Journal of Obstetrics and Gynecology* 196:186.e1–186.e5.

Flemming DD, Scott JF (2004) The informed consent doctrine: what veterinarians should tell their clients. *Journal of the American Veterinary Medical Association* 224(9):1436–1439.

Gafni A, Charles C, Whelan T (1998) The physician–patient encounter: the physician as a perfect agent for the patient versus the informed treatment decision-making model. *Social Science and Medicine* 47(3):347–354.

General Medical Council (1998) *Seeking Patients' Consent: The Ethical Considerations.* GMC, London.

Ginsburg ME, Kravitz RL, Sandberg WA (2000) A survey of physician attitudes and practices concerning cost-effectiveness in patient care. *Western Journal of Medicine* 173(6):390–394.

Goldblatt D (2006) Patient–physician communication using consent forms. *Archives of Surgery* 141:715.

Gray C, Eaves RE, Walsh SJ, Wilson CJ (2005) A final year special study module in veterinary communication skills. *Association for Medical Education in Europe Conference Abstracts 2005*, AMEE, Dundee, p. 188.

Klein WMP, Stefanek ME (2007) Cancer risk elicitation and communication: lessons from the psychology of risk perception. *CA Cancer Journal for Clinicians* 57:147–167.

Lashley M, Talley W, Lands LC, Keyserlingk, EW (2000) Informed proxy consent: communication between pediatric surgeons and surrogates about surgery. *Pediatrics* 105:591–597.

Levinson W, Kao A, Kuby A, Thisted RA (2005) Not all patients want to participate in decision-making. *Journal of General Internal Medicine* 20:531–535.

Lill MM, Wilkinson TJ (2005) Judging a book by its cover: descriptive survey of patients' preferences for doctors' appearance and mode of address. *British Medical Journal* 331:1524–1527.

Makoul G, Zick A, Green M (2007) An evidence-based perspective on greetings in medical encounters. *Archives of Internal Medicine* 167:1172–1176.

Matlack CB (2004) More on the sentient property debate. *Journal of the American Veterinary Medical Association* 225(10):1526–1527.

Ness M (2002) Decision making in the management of severe limb trauma. *In Practice* 24:302–309.

Palmboom GG, Willems DL, Janssen NBAT, de Haes JCJM (2007) Doctors' views on disclosing or withholding information on low risks of complications. *Journal of Medical Ethics* 33:67–70.

Pullen S (2006) Research on people: ethical considerations. In: Pullen S, Gray C (eds), *Ethics, Law and the Veterinary Nurse.* Elsevier, Edinburgh.

Rehman SU, Nietert PJ, Cope DW, Osborne Kilpatrick A (2005) What to wear today? Effect of doctor's attire on the trust and confidence of patients. *American Journal of Medicine* 118(11):1279–1286.

Rollin BE (2006) Euthanasia and quality of life. *Journal of the American Veterinary Medical Association* 228(7):1014–1016.

Royal College of Veterinary Surgeons (2008a) *Guide to Professional Conduct.* RCVS, London.

Royal College of Veterinary Surgeons (2008b) Guide to professional conduct Part 3 Annexes e: communication and consent. Available online: http://www.rcvs.org.uk/Templates/PreviousNext.asp?NodeID=89767&int2ndParentNodeID=89738&int1stParentNodeID=89642 (accessed 31 May 2009).

Royal College of Veterinary Surgeons (2008c) Suggested consent form for euthanasia. Available online: http://www.rcvs.org.uk/Templates/PreviousNext.asp?NodeID=89767&int2ndParentNodeID=89738&int1stParentNodeID=89642 (accessed 31 May 2009).

Royal College of Veterinary Surgeons (2009) Suggested form of consent for anaesthesia and surgery. Available online: http://www.rcvs.org.uk/Templates/PreviousNext.asp?NodeID=89767&int2ndParentNodeID=89738&int1stParentNodeID=89642 (accessed 4 September 2009).

Schloendorff vs Society of New York Hospital (1914) 211 N.Y. 125, 105 N.E. 92.

Shen J, Andersen R, Brook R, Kominski G, Albert PS, Wenger N (2004) The effect of payment method on clinical decision-making. *Medical Care* 42(3):297–302.

Sokol DK (2007) Can deceiving patients be morally acceptable? *British Medical Journal* 334:984–986.

Timmermans D, Molewijk B, Stiggelbout A, Kievit J (2004) Different formats for communicating surgical risks to patients and the effect on choice of treatment. *Patient Education and Counseling* 54:255–263.

Trevana LJ, Davey HM, Barratt A, Butow P, Caldwell P (2006) A systematic review on communicating with patients about evidence. *Journal of Evaluation in Clinical Practice* 12(1):13–23.

Wiggins MN, Coker K, Hicks EK (2009) Patient perceptions of professionalism: implications for residency education. *Medical Education* 43:28–33.

Wojciechowska JI, Hewson CJ, Stryhn H, Guy NC, Patronek GJ, Timmons V (2005) Development of a discriminative questionnaire to assess nonphysical aspects of the quality of life of dogs. *American Journal of Veterinary Research* 66(8):1453–1460.

Wright M (1995) Consent forms – a necessary evil. *In Practice* 17:482–484.

Compassionate communication: working with grief

Susan Elizabeth Dawson

Introduction

Working in veterinary medicine and animal welfare presents specific and complex challenges, not least because of the extremes and intensity of human emotions encountered and experienced at times of crisis and loss. Compassionate communication enables a fusion of genuine care and professionalism, facilitating development of trusting working partnerships between professionals and owners, that brings about a greater depth of understanding of the individual relationships between people and their pets – the human–companion animal bond (HCAB).

Whilst the HCAB is not a new concept, understanding of human emotions arising as a consequence of 'the bond' is relatively recent. The relevance of this is particularly pertinent to the veterinary profession and animal welfare organizations because of the existence of the option of active euthanasia, which gives rise to a distinct category of loss (Dawson 2007a). The unique type of human grief resulting from owners' direct personal responsibility for the death of their companion animal by euthanasia is known as *responsibility grief* (Dawson 2007a). Veterinary and other animal welfare professionals too may also experience a type of professional *responsibility grief* directly linked to repeated and sustained professional responsibility for, and exposure to, euthanasia (Dawson 2007a). Within practice, responsibility grief requires recognition, sensitive management and specific approaches to emotional support.

Human emotional responses to a range of companion animal welfare issues, e.g. compliance with treatment protocols, pet obesity, palliative treatment and care, are all further complicated by the ambiguous status of companion animals in society. Current research, however, firmly shows that most people perceive and relate pets as valued family members (Barton Ross & Baron-Sorensen 2007; Cohen 2002; Dawson 2006, 2007a, 2007b), but despite this, emotions associated with human–animal relationships are often dismissed as sentimental, ridiculous or even pathological. Consequently, pet owners can be left with little or no support from others, including close family members, and as a result naturally turn to the veterinary profession for understanding, validation and emotional support in response to multiple situations arising as a consequence of the HCAB.

This chapter provides a brief outline of what the HCAB is and explores key practical skills and interventions, enabling compassionate communication, facilitating more sensitive working with human emotions encountered in practice. As a fundamental basis for enabling in-practice provision of client-centred emotional support, the concept of *bond-centred veterinary practice* (BCVP) is introduced, locating straightforward practical steps facilitating a bond-centred approach to working with human emotions including the following:

- An insight into the relevance of the HCAB in veterinary practice.
- How to recognize human emotions arising from the bond, including responsibility grief (Dawson 2007a).
- BCVP principles incorporating development of emotional support protocols, facilitation of bond-centred euthanasia practice and an emotion-friendly environment.
- Compassionate communication skills for responding to the emotional needs arising from HCAB, including applied use of illness trajectory mapping (Dawson 2007a) as a clinical communication tool, facilitating review of quality-of-life indicators during palliative care.
- Practical solutions for provision of on-site emotional support, including continuing care (palliative care) and bereavement clinics, incorporating an outline of considerations for setting up and running a pet loss support group.

A continuum of human emotions is encountered in practice ranging from the shock, numbness and denial at receiving a terminal prognosis, to the deep and very real distress of requesting and witnessing the death of a loved companion animal at the time of euthanasia. No two clients are the same; adopting a bond-centred approach to working with human emotions essentially involves taking a holistic perspective in trying to gain an understanding of the client in the wider context of their life-world and circumstances. This means responding sensitively to specific animal welfare needs, whilst taking into account the relationship between the pet and the person. To be able to do this effectively within clinical practice involves gaining a richer understanding and insight into the HCAB.

THE HCAB

The HCAB is what ultimately motivates owners to seek out veterinary care for companion animals. The AVMA (American Veterinary Medical Association) provides a statement defining the HCAB (which in the USA is referred to as the human–animal bond – HAB), locating its relevance at the heart of veterinary practice:

> The human-animal bond is a mutually beneficial and dynamic relationship between people and animals that is influenced by behaviours that are essential to the health and well being of both. This includes but is not limited to emotional, psychological and physical interactions of people, animals and the environment. The veterinarian's role in the human-animal bond is to maximize potentials of this relationship between people and animals (AVMA 2006).

The AVMA further recognizes the following:

- The existence of the HAB and its importance to the client and community health
- The HAB has existed for thousands of years
- The HAB has major significance for veterinary medicine because, as veterinary medicine serves society, it fulfils both human and animal needs (AVMA 2006)

In the UK, the human–pet bond is generally referred to as the HCAB, whereas in the USA HAB is the preferred term for all human–animal relationships and interactions, including those with companion animals (Dawson et al. 2007). The language used to talk about pets and pet-keeping has evolved, particularly over the past decade, reflecting the change in status of companion animals as legitimate family members (Cohen 2002; Dawson 2006, 2007a). The preferred term now used by animal welfare professionals is *companion animal*, which recognizes the mutuality of the relationship (Lagoni et al. 1994), whereas the term *pet* is more frequently associated with 'ownership'. Within this chapter, these two terms are used interchangeably in recognition of this evolution over time. Falls in human birth rates in the Western world and increased social mobility have been given as possible reasons for the increased popularity of companion animals as an alternative choice of family structure (Barton Ross & Baron-Sorensen 2007; Dawson 2007a). It is, therefore, not surprising that human emotions traditionally more exclusively associated with human–human relationships are also present as a consequence of the HCAB.

There are a number of scientific theories applied for understanding the HCAB that can help shed light on the human emotions arising as a consequence of the bond. Traditionally, Wilson's (1993) *biophilia* hypothesis has been applied for understanding more generic human–animal interactions, that is the HCAB. This theory states that people have a natural affinity with other living things, both plants and animals: 'Biophilia if it exists, and I believe it exists, is the innately emotional affiliation of human beings with organisms' (Wilson 1993). Biophilia could explain the natural human fascination and need for contact with other animals that some people experience, but does not provide a basis for unravelling and understanding the more intricate personal facets of the HCAB. It is these facets that most commonly give rise to the strong emotions encountered in practice, such as love.

'Many people openly and enthusiastically admit to loving their pets' (Crawford et al. 2006). As a result, it is not surprising that theories of human–human attachment are most usually applied to explicate the HCAB. Bowlby's *attachment theory* (1969, 1979, 1980, 1988) is frequently applied in understanding the strong affectional ties between people and their pets (Beetz 2007). Attachment theory is rooted in an evolutionary understanding of the HCAB and studies investigating mother–child relationships (Bowlby 1969). Characteristics associated with attachment include seeking proximity, distress at separation, pleasure at reunion and general orientation to the primary caregiver.

The purposes of attachment are safety, provision of a secure base (emotionally safe place), anxiety reduction and promoting emotional and self-development. When a human–companion animal attachment is threatened or lost, the animal is grieved for as an individual, perceived as possessing unique characteristics that have often been described, by owners, as being a personality (Dawson 2007a). It is understandable that at a time of loss or threat of loss/trauma within the bond, owners naturally experience a range of emotions comparable to, or sometimes surpassing, that of human–human attachments. It is the depth and quality of a relationship that shapes the intensity of the grief experienced when the relationship is lost. Understanding the nature of the person–pet attachment can enable *empathic responding* from the veterinary team and a greater understanding of the *relational value* of the companion animal in the owner's life-world.

Current researchers investigating the HCAB (Brown 2004a, 2004b; Dawson 2007a) have explored the relational value of companion animals in the lives of their owners, investigating how owners experience the qualities provided by the relationship with their companion animal. This gives insight into the function of the pet, such as surrogate, social lubricant/facilitator or friend. Companion animals can provide vital functions in the life-world of their owners (Brown 2004a; Dawson 2007a) – which are known as self-object functions in self-psychology (Kohut 1971), a branch of psychology grounded in psychodynamic theory. Owners' experiences of these functions possess characteristics and qualities likened to those of key human relationships:

- *Parent–child* – In providing opportunities to care and be responsible for the companion animal.
- *Child–parent* – Whereby the companion animal's presence provides feelings of security and comfort for owners.
- *Sibling–sibling* – Through generating opportunities for play and fun, companion animal likened to 'kid brother or sister' in that owners feel responsible for the welfare and well-being of their pet.
- *Advocate–best friend* – A relationship of equality/partnership in which owners assume the role of advocate at times of need for the companion animal (Dawson 2007a).

Companion animals play important roles in the lives of people, as attachment beings and relational partners. It is therefore understandable that when it comes to their welfare and care, human emotions will be integral within this process.

Facets of the HCAB

In order to be able to recognize and respond to the specific human needs and emotions arising as a consequence of the HCAB, it is essential to gain an understanding of the individual facets (qualities) that contribute to building the bond between pets and people. This can be further relevant in enabling compassionate communication at times of crisis and loss, diffusing and deflecting emotions in conflict situations, encouraging compliance with treatment protocols, facilitating joint review of quality-of-life indicators during palliative treatment and care, developing a bond between owners and the practice team based on mutual trust and encouragement and maintaining client loyalty to the practice.

Recent research (Dawson 2007a), investigating human–companion animal relationships in the UK has identified what has become known as the *facets of the HCAB*, essentially revealing the 'ingredients' that can make up a close human–companion animal relationship:

- *Exclusivity* – A sense of having a 'special' bond with, being chosen/preferred by a companion animal.
- *Caring, nurturing role* – This included rescuing animals and the nurturing of young animals.
- *Personality/perceived individuality of the companion animal* – Experienced and related to as individual, irreplaceable and unique and possessing a 'personality'.

- *Perceived reciprocity* – Involving talking to a companion animal, mutual trust and non-sexual love.
- *Companion animal family member status* – This extends to the use of human familial metaphors to describe human–companion animal relationships, e.g. like a brother/sister, like a child or surrogate parent (further revealing the relational qualities experienced by owners).
- *Duration of time spent together* – Length of ownership, amount of time spent together during the day and night.
- *Proximity* (emotional and physical) – A sense of closeness, sustained need for actual physical proximity of the companion animal.
- *Compatibility* – With the caregiver's personality (either complementary or similar), appearance and behaviour (Dawson 2007a).

Active awareness and understanding of the facets of the HCAB enable greater ability to recognize and respond to human emotions arising from particular facets of the bond; for example, a client may be deeply distressed that their pet died during the surgery without them being present at the time. The origin of this distress could be located in the perceived mutual trust owners feel they share with their companion animals and a sustained need for proximity. Verbally acknowledging this as being 'normal' within an attachment relationship can help validate owners' feelings and enable understanding of their origins. Similarly, there is a natural tendency for some owners to anthropomorphize companion animals, such as giving pets human-like characteristics and traits. 'Human emotions and behaviours are thus often attributed to animals despite the fact that little or no scientific evidence exists to support the presence of such characteristics' (Lagoni et al. 1994). It can be easy, as a professional exposed to crisis situations on a daily basis, to lose sight of the *personal* factors and *context* that construct owners' emotional responses that could be linked to anthropomorphism. These reactions may then be perceived as exaggerated, abnormal or even hysterical if taken out of context, when in actual fact these are simply normal, natural consequences of the bond. Verbally acknowledging the conferred personhood that some owners bestow onto their companion animals can be helpful in reflecting back specific aspects of the relationship, enabling a greater self-understanding of these associated emotions. Having briefly explored what the HCAB is, it becomes obvious that human emotions are an integral part of people–pet relationships. It is helpful at this point to explain more fully what emotions are.

Human emotions

The word 'emotion' comes from the Latin meaning to move, excite, stir up or agitate. Stratton and Hayes (1999) define emotion as 'the experience of subjective feelings which have a positive or negative value for the individual'. Emotional responses possess different components, known widely by psychologists as the ABC:

- Affective – *Feelings*, for example joy, fear and anger.
- Behavioural – *Movements or actions* a person performs (voluntary and involuntary), for example, increased heart rate and muscle tension, shouting, which could be associated with feelings of anger.
- Cognitive – *Thinking*, decision making, reason.

Emotions usually arise spontaneously rather than through a conscious process and are often involuntary (outside conscious control). Pet owners' felt and expressed emotions will be related to personal feelings; perceptions and beliefs; relationships between beliefs and feelings that may involve past experiences (both the animal and the human); elements from reality and imagination; culture, religion, age, gender and social class.

Our own culture and life experience with companion animals may also lead to making assumptions about which emotions are 'right' and 'normal' to feel and express about our relationship with pets. Frequently observed and encountered emotions in veterinary and animal welfare charity practice will now be examined from a bond-centred perspective.

There are widely recognized human emotions associated with attachment to a companion animal:

- *Anticipation/excitement* – Linked with newly acquired/adopted/rescued animals.
- *Grief* – This is the reaction to loss or threat of loss; it is a normal reaction for people attached to their companion animals and can be manifested behaviourally (e.g. crying), psychologically (e.g. feelings of depression), cognitively (e.g. thoughts of blame) and physically (e.g. insomnia and vomiting).
- *Happiness* – Generates a sense of cohesion between people and pets and is often contagious to others.
- *Joy* – Obvious in facial expression, lots of smiles and laughter.
- *Love* – Could be verbally articulated openly in the surgery, may be visibly expressed by lots of tactile contact and could also be associated with feelings of embarrassment in some people.
- *Pride* – May be linked to a working animal, assistance animal partnership or 'show' animals.
- *Responsibility* – Expressed in nurturing, caring and rescuing behaviours; can be recognized through information seeking about welfare issues, intent listening during consults and meticulous compliance with treatment protocols.
- *Security* – Some owners may gain their sense of security from the presence of/interactions with their companion animal and could present in a reluctance to leave the companion animal at the practice without them being present; signs of hyperattachment and overt distress at the possibility of separation or threatened loss; may be explicitly tactile with the animal; seeking emotional and physical proximity.
- *Trust* (usually perceived as two-way interaction between people and pets) – Owners may talk to their companion animal, providing a verbal explanation/commentary of events in a consult; may result in a desire to oversee/be involved in consultation examinations; reluctance to leave companion animal in the surgery without being there; attention to ensuring the animal appears calm with no outward signs of visible discomfort or distress.

Positive human emotions often feel easy to be in the presence of and can be contagious to others, creating feelings of optimism, whereas it can feel difficult to be in the presence of hostile and more negative human emotions such as anger or distress. *Self-awareness* in practice enables reflection on the origin of our own moods, helping us to identify if we have been contaminated by the emotions of others. It also enables identification of possible prejudices grounded in our own past experiences and personal belief systems. This can be particularly important when working in highly emotionally charged and distressing situations, such as at times of loss.

An inevitable consequence of attachment is grief on separation and loss. 'Love and loss are two sides of the same coin, we cannot have one without risking the other' (Parkes 2006). When the HCAB is broken, lost or under threat of loss, owners and veterinary team members experience loss. 'Loss is defined as an ending or as a point of change and transition' (Lagoni et al. 1994). It can be helpful to be familiar with the different types of loss that may be encountered in veterinary practice.

Types of loss

Bereavement refers to the loss of a significant other. Grief is the term used to describe reactions to loss. Companion animal death is only one type of loss. Relinquishment, such as due to relocation or owner's ill health, theft, pets straying or going missing are all further examples of companion animal loss giving rise to bereavement. Lagoni et al. (1994) identify understanding of four types of loss as being pertinent to the veterinary profession:

1. Primary loss
2. Secondary loss
3. Ambiguous loss
4. Symbolic loss

Primary loss

Primary loss is the loss of the actual companion animal, for example where the death of owner's pet is the main origin of their grief. The animal is perceived as intrinsically valuable and missed in its own right.

Secondary loss

Secondary losses are the associated disruptions and stresses caused by the primary loss. These losses tend to focus more on the relational value of animals in the life of their owners and have the greatest impact on those who rely on their pets for their only source of social support, companionship, motivation and purpose. Other important and often overlooked secondary losses can be the loss of the caring relationship with the veterinary team, and the discontinuation of regular visits to the surgery, which could provide the only opportunity for extended contact with others (e.g. for some older people).

Ambiguous loss

These types of losses leave questions in owners' minds, for example, the whereabouts of a pet, in the case of a missing or stolen animal or where the causes of death remain unknown. Feelings of confusion, incompletion and a relentless need to gather further information about the circumstances of the loss are characteristic within grieving patterns. Actively, verbally acknowledging the stress and turmoil that ambiguous loss brings about is important for the caregiver as it normalizes often very uncomfortable, chaotic feelings. Providing practical information, such as the contact details for The Missing Pets Bureau and The Blue Cross/SCAS Pet Bereavement Support Service (PBSS), can provide further validation of feelings of grief, as well as much-needed access to practical help and support. It is essential to validate feelings of grief as being normal.

Symbolic loss

Companion animals may represent a link with earlier/other losses in someone's life. This may be a last link to a deceased spouse, friend or a special place or time of life that has now ended. The loss of the pet removes the final connection. Although the companion animal loss is significant in and as itself, the grief experienced may be intensified when past losses are grieved in parallel to the existing loss. Verbally acknowledging and validating this intensification can be helpful. Sensitive referral to an external agency working with human losses, such as Cruse Bereavement Care, helps to make clear the limitations of support that can be provided by the practice. Referral information should include website and helpline numbers. Suggestions can also be made to seek referral for counselling via their general practitioner.

Provision of nurse-facilitated bereavement clinics and on-site pet loss support groups can enable an emotionally supported transition through the different types of loss associated with pet bereavement, providing space to remember the relationship that has been lost with understanding compassionate others. These practical interventions for supporting grieving clients are described more fully later in this chapter. To be able to provide effective support essentially involves having awareness and understanding of human emotions associated with grief.

Grief and companion animal loss

Grief is the reaction to loss. Frequently encountered human emotions associated with companion animal loss include feelings of abandonment, anger, confusion, denial, depression, doubt, fear, guilt, numbness, regret, relief, responsibility, sadness, shock and searching.

Feelings of abandonment occur where companion animals have provided 'parental' qualities in their owners' life; for example, a sense of security, acceptance and comfort, and could involve intensified feelings if the owner perceives the veterinary team have not been supportive before, during and immediately after the loss. Providing options for structured bereavement support, for example nurse-facilitated bereavement clinics, on-site pet loss support group or enabling access to external organizations such as The Blue Cross/SCAS PBSS can help generate a sense of a more supported transition for owners.

Anger may be directed at self, other family members, veterinary professionals involved in caring for the animal or even the pet for dying, and can be expressed behaviourally (externalized) through shouting, swearing, becoming physically abusive and violent to others or (internalized) directed inwards towards self, which may involve self-punishing behaviour, feelings of deep frustration and self-loathing. In extreme cases it could result in self-harm: alcohol abuse or self-cutting. Anger is a natural response to distress and/or challenge for some people. There may be situations where the anger is actually valid, for example, when an animal is involved in a road traffic accident because someone left the gate open or instances of medical negligence/error. An important first step in working with more hostile emotions is to allow owners to have their say, followed by verbally acknowledging feelings of anger: 'It sounds like you're very frustrated with Sooty's illness, it's difficult waiting for a diagnosis.'

Confusion is closely linked to shock and denial. Owners may find it difficult, if not impossible, to absorb and understand clinical information at times of distress. This requires careful and patient re-explanations of information. Clarification with written information sheets can be useful. Provision of the option of nurse-facilitated clinics (palliative/continuing care clinics) can be valuable in providing further clarification and re-explanation of clinical information and treatment protocols, enabling extended opportunities for owners to ask questions, helping to eliminate and lessen confusion associated with stressful situations such as anticipated illness trajectory or treatment protocols.

Denial often originates from unconscious and subconscious needs for self-protection. Owners may carry on exactly as before a diagnosis/prognosis or a loss. This can result in veterinary professionals feeling frustration, annoyance, impatience and sometimes outright anger towards owners, particularly in terms of lack of compliance with treatment protocols such as weight management programmes. At a time of terminal prognosis, denial may present as an apparent lack of response or anticipated reaction. Denial can function as what is known as a *psychological defence mechanism*, that is, a strategy put into place to protect self. Helping owners accept the reality of the situation involves patience and sensitivity, being congruent (saying what is felt) and attempting to make information more concrete, for example, by reinforcing through supplementary written material, practical visible examples. Encouraging owners to talk about the situation can be facilitated by repetition of information and through the use of open questions; for example, 'What practical information do you need from me that might help you feel better able to cope with Spike's heart murmur?'

Depression is a much misused term in describing feelings of deep sadness. True depression involves a reduced state of both psychological and physiological functioning, such that it impairs everyday life. Common symptoms are loss of interest and inability to enjoy experiences, sadness, loss of appetite, sleep disturbances (especially in the early hours), passivity, suicidal thoughts or intentions – although very severe depressions may involve only a few of these symptoms (Stratton & Hayes 1999). Depressed owners, when encountered, may be apathetic towards treatment advice, unable to comply with protocols and may require help from a human mental health professional, for example, a community psychiatric nurse or social worker. Some owners may react to the loss of their companion animal by becoming depressed. Providing ongoing support for truly depressed owners is outside the remit and scope of emotional support provision within veterinary practice and may require sensitive referral to their family doctor, community psychiatric nurse or social worker – this can only be done after discussion with a client directly and with their full informed consent if the referral is made by the practice, in order to protect client confidentiality and ensure adherence to the professional code of ethics.

For a client deeply attached to their pet, uncertainty related to euthanasia decision making, particularly retrospectively, is frequently encountered. Doubt is a natural and normal part of euthanasia-related responsibility grief (Dawson 2007a). It can result in a need to exhaustively re-visit the euthanasia decision-making process in an effort to clearly identify a selfless and sound clinical basis for the euthanasia decision, in order to reduce feelings of guilt, which are directly associated with responsibility for the death. Allowing time pre-euthanasia for discussion and review of the illness trajectory, discussion of personally important facets of the bond, illuminating both subjective as well as clinical quality-of-life indicators within a continuing (palliative) care clinic, can be very helpful in lessening or eliminating feelings of doubt post-euthanasia. In this way, feelings of lingering guilt may be lessened for owners.

Some owners can experience fear in relation to illness trajectories, their ability to care for a terminally ill companion animal, witnessing deterioration and decline of a loved pet, requesting and witnessing the euthanasia event and imagining what their companion animal may experience at the time of death. It is crucial to remember that owners may be unfamiliar with the euthanasia procedure and because of this they could conjure up imagined horrors, which leave them traumatized. Fear can be linked to thoughts about the companion animal, perceiving or knowing what is going to happen at the time of euthanasia (anticipation of their own death). This can raise some intense feelings of regret, betrayed trust, guilt and doubt in relation to the appropriateness of the timing and the decision itself (Dawson 2007a). Allowing enough time pre-euthanasia to explain and clarify detailed information relating to the course of a disease process and the process of euthanasia is a key in managing owners' fear in relation to end-of-life care for a terminally ill pet.

Integrally linked with owners' personal responsibility for the euthanasia of their companion animal, feelings of guilt may complicate the grieving process and result in a need to find someone to blame. Usually, this blame is internally directed (self blame), but it can also result in blaming the veterinary team responsible for the care of the companion animal and the euthanasia event itself. In some instances where the euthanasia has been more complicated, for example, difficulty finding and raising a vein, or a dog becoming aggressive towards the vet/nurse during a home euthanasia and struggling just before death, members of the veterinary team may also experience feelings of guilt, which are linked directly to professional responsibility. Bringing these feelings into conscious awareness and recognizing them as normal reactions is the first step in learning to work effectively with these more challenging emotions in self and others.

Numbness is closely associated with denial and may present behaviourally in owners being uncommunicative. Outwardly, they may appear uncompassionate, uncaring and unmoved by events. This can result in a misconstrual that the owner does not care about the pet and provoke feelings of rising antagonism in veterinary teams, with a tendency to judge owners unfavourably. Knowing that people respond individually and differently to potentially stressful or traumatic events should enable veterinary professionals to be accepting of reactions that may appear initially strange or out of context. Communicating this acceptance to owners is essential within an empathic relationship.

Feelings of regret could be linked to accidental death and a sense of responsibility for this which could be actual or perceived, failure to adhere to treatment protocols, inability to leave a violent partner who threatened to kill a loved companion animal; most usually, feelings of regret are associated with euthanasia retrospectively and can be in relation to the timing of the euthanasia (perceived as being too soon/waited too long), how the procedure progressed, not having been present. Interestingly, there are few reports of feelings of regret at being present. In fact, remaining with an animal at the time of euthanasia may actually function as a protective factor in enabling a sense of continuing care, trust in the euthanasia decision and in enabling knowledge of what actually happened at the time of death (Dawson 2007a). Wherever possible, owners should be encouraged and actively supported to enable them to stay with their companion animal.

Relief can be accompanied by feelings of guilt as owners perceive it to be wrong to feel relieved; relief may be openly expressed by tears or other behavioural responses that could be construed as being more inappropriate, such as smiling, laughter or an open verbal declaration of relief at being freed from long-term caring commitments. It is essential not to judge owners and to communicate acceptance of their feelings.

Responsibility is often confused with feelings of guilt in relation to euthanasia; owners are enabled to accept personal responsibility for the care and welfare of their companion animals including direct responsibility for euthanasia, and actually appear to be more emotionally robust in coping with the loss of a companion animal. Responsibility needs to be positively framed highlighting its centrality within the HCAB and animal welfare. The professional responsibility of the veterinary team for informing the euthanasia decision through provision of clinical information, review and assessment along with responsibility for the actual euthanasia procedure must be made visible to owners enabling a sense of shared responsibility for the death of their companion animal.

People grieve individually, but sadness is often recognizable through behaviour, for example, crying, sobbing, becoming quiet and withdrawn, looking miserable, lack of interest in activities once enjoyed and increased pessimism. Unlike depression, sadness usually lasts for a shorter duration of time, is not as intense and does not significantly impair everyday function or require medical intervention.

Shock is linked to numbness and denial; people in shock may look visibly dismayed and ask lots of questions, becoming 'information hungry' in an effort to process events or alternatively may temporarily shut down, be unable to take in information and appear to withdraw.

Observed across species as a symptom of grief, it is not uncommon for someone who has experienced a loss to search for the lost object; for example, owners may repeatedly come back to the surgery on the day and time of the death, subconsciously searching for the deceased pet. In instances of ambiguous loss, where pets have gone missing, some owners may spend literally hundreds of hours and pounds searching for the lost animal; a few owners have reported physically wandering, engaging in actual searching behaviour, calling out the name of the pet after it has died and, whilst cognitively knowing it is not possible to see/be reunited with the deceased animal, experiencing a compelling urge to search and relocate the deceased (Dawson 2007a).

Grief is a universal human experience, a natural and spontaneous reaction to loss (Lagoni et al. 1994) and is the personal process of adjustment to loss. It is not an event, or a predictable, linear journey. What is usually understood as being 'normal grief' is not time limited; it may last for days, weeks, months or even years, depending on the personal significance of the relationship that has been lost. Grieving involves a continuum of emotions from feelings of being able to cope with thoughts of being overwhelmed and temporarily suicidal. Grief does not go away, but rather lessens in its intensity and rawness with the passage of time as it moves from being at the centre of conscious awareness to partly inhabiting the subconscious, until brought back into immediate consciousness through triggers and reminders. The range of reactions experienced within what is frequently understood to be 'normal grief' is shown in Table 4.1.

It is essential to understand though that grief does not just occur at the time of actual loss, but can begin beforehand in anticipation of what is to come. This type of grief is known as *anticipatory grief* (Rando 1986).

Table 4.1   The range of reactions experienced within what is frequently understood to be 'normal grief'

Physical Reactions	Cognitive (Thinking)
Insomnia – not sleeping	Blame – self, vet, others including the animal for getting ill
Crying	Information seeking – about the medical condition
Diarrhoea/vomiting	Thinking about the animal and talking about the animal
Tiredness	'processing out'
Lack of concentration	Reliving the event of the death
Somatizing – physical symptoms similar to the deceased animal	

Emotional/Psychological	Social
Sadness	Temporary increased dependency or withdrawal from human others
Depression – extreme and overwhelming sadness	Feeling isolated and alone
Shock	Loss of identity as an animal caregiver
Denial	Need to take some time off work
Guilt	

From Dawson and Campbell (2005) and Stewart (1999).

Anticipatory grief

Recent research (Dawson 2007a) has revealed that a process of anticipatory grieving for companion animals may begin at the first visible onset of disease or decline or at the time of terminal prognosis by the veterinary surgeon. Grief can begin when there is a threat of loss or of disruption of the bond. This is known as anticipatory grieving (Rando 1986) and is frequently encountered in relation to the HCAB and veterinary practice. It can involve the following:

- Denial, shock, avoidance of reality
- Panic, anxiety – sometimes inhibiting ability to listen to information being given and to follow instructions
- Information-seeking behaviour (about the disease process, anticipated trajectory) or paradoxical denial
- Hypervigilance – close observation, anxious watching of the companion animal
- Rumination on the causes/course of a disease
- Rehearsing the euthanasia decision-making process
- Rehearsing the death and its consequences (anticipating the personal impact of both primary and secondary losses)
- Meticulous reviewing of quality-of-life indicators
- Feelings of deep sadness, tearfulness, being unable to cope
- Insomnia, interrupted sleep through night-time care-giving to sick companion animals
- Practical preparation for the death event and after-death body care, for example visiting pet crematorium and choosing pet cemetery plot (Dawson 2007a)

Meyers (2000) notes that there is no socially sanctioned or accepted way of dealing with anticipatory grief over a dying companion animal and as a result it is often dealt with by premature euthanasia.

Excruciating grief is quickly put an end to with logic, rationale and well-meaning advice of friends, family or insensitive professionals who make comments such as 'Why put her through it? He is 14 years old after all ...' (Meyers 2000).

When owners lack knowledge of alternatives available and have no previous experience of providing end-of-life care for a companion animal, euthanasia is often turned to as a way of relieving perceived pain and of preventing future pain, without taking into account the actual disease process and illness trajectory, and available medication/treatment to manage this effectively. Sensitive, clear information about options and choices provided in a warm, empathic, supportive environment can enable informed decision making. This includes a review of subjective as well as clinical quality-of-life indicators through the use of illness trajectory mapping (Dawson 2007a) within continuing (palliative) care clinics with owners. Illness trajectory mapping can be used as a clinical communication tool to enable support-ive management of emotions associated with anticipatory grief (Dawson 2007a), essentially involving owners in the process and creating a sense of empowerment. Being able to put a name to the uncomfortable feelings of anticipatory grief can also be very helpful for a major-ity of people; for example, 'These feelings that you are experiencing are normal – it's what is called anticipatory grief, this is a way of preparing yourself for what is to come at a later stage through rehearsing possibilities. I'm wondering what information can I give you that could be useful?'

Clarifying owners' understanding about the anticipated course of a disease process is es-sential in enabling management of anxiety within anticipatory grief. It is common for owners to feel powerless at the time of terminal diagnosis/prognosis. In gaining information about what can be expected to happen, it enables greater preparation and identification of what actions are needed to ensure the comfort of their pet, for example, compliance with admin-istering medication, following a special diet, and weight reduction. Assuming responsibil-ity for what it is possible to control re-affirms owners as active agents for the continued welfare and protection of their pet, which is essential in retaining their role and reinforc-ing their identity as primary caregivers. Whilst re-affirming and making visible owners' re-sponsibility for their pets are vitally important, it is necessary to understand that the sense of personal responsibility evoked from the euthanasia decision leads to a unique type of grieving found almost exclusively within veterinary medicine – responsibility grief (Dawson 2007a).

Responsibility grief

Companion animal euthanasia has been revealed as being a distinct category of loss, in that owners have direct personal responsibility for the death of their companion animal (Dawson 2007a). Veterinary professionals have responsibility for clearly communicating clinical infor-mation to help inform euthanasia decision making and for the actual euthanasia procedure. The practice of active euthanasia is almost exclusive to veterinary medicine, as human eu-thanasia is illegal in most of the world. Despite hopes that pets will die natural deaths, eu-thanasia remains the major agent of death for companion animals in the Western world.

Companion animal euthanasia results in the unique type of grief known as responsibility grief (Dawson 2007a), which possesses the following characteristics:

- The presence of direct personal responsibility for requesting the intentional death of another living being for whom one has care-giving/guardianship responsibility.
- A period of anticipatory grief (experienced before the death, involving feelings of anxiety in rehearsing the possible death scenarios and the potential feelings arising from having direct personal responsibility for the death, by active euthanasia).
- Feelings of impotence and powerlessness over the illness and anticipated illness trajectory.
- Reviewing of subjective quality-of-life indicators in an effort to locate pivotal (final deciding) and key (contributory) moments informing euthanasia decision making.
- A dynamic, psycho-ethical dialectic (sort of a conversation with self/internal dialogue) of personally construed opposite emotions and thoughts, integral within this are interchangeable feelings of responsibility and guilt; doubt is usually present in relation to the timing, appropriateness of choice and motivation (altruistic or egoistic) for the euthanasia.
- Feeling of disenfranchisement, i.e. being alone and unrecognized as a legitimate griever coexisting alongside feelings that the relationship itself (the HCAB) is unrecognized as significant by others, fear of minimization of the loss (by others), personal ridicule and judgement. A sense of having to keep both the significance of the relationship and the gravity of the loss secret, further complicated by paradoxical feelings associated with having requested the death – by euthanasia.

Animal welfare professionals may also experience a type of professional responsibility grief (Dawson 2007a) arising from emotions associated with repeated exposure to, and responsibility for, multiple euthanasias. It is essential within emotional support protocols that pathways for staff to access support are made explicit, for example, through employee assistance programmes, buddying systems at work, the Vetlife website and telephone helpline, or access to private counselling. The characteristics of professional responsibility grief include the following:

- The presence of direct professional responsibility for the intentional death of another living being under one's professional care.
- Rumination over clinical decision making, past euthanasia procedures.
- Negative anticipation of future euthanasias.
- Anxiety and dread related to euthanasia decision making.
- Anxiety and unease arising from the sense of powerfulness evoked from actively ending life; fear of the potential for abuse of this power.
- A psycho-ethical dialectic (dialogue with self), integral within this process involving interchangeable feelings of self-exoneration and self-persecution related to responsibility for multiple deaths by euthanasia.
- Feelings of disenfranchisement arising from a sense of having to keep personal emotions hidden and secret for fear of being accused of being unprofessional, incompetent and unstable and of reprisals from this in the workplace.

Figure 4.1 illuminates the coexistence of strong contradictory emotions within a dual process through which owners try to locate evidence of altruistic (genuine, other-centred) decision

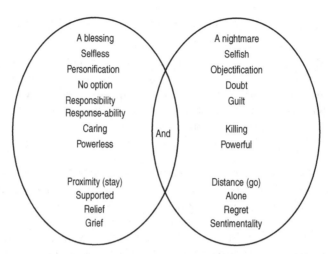

Figure 4.1 The dialectics of responsibility grief (Dawson 2007a): an intrapersonal dialectic of coexisting contradictory thoughts and emotions.

making and motivation for the euthanasia. Owners' very sense of self (as a loving, caring person) can be temporarily, sometimes permanently, threatened or lost as a result of feelings of guilt and doubt in relation to the timing of and motivation for the euthanasia. Compassionate communication when working with people experiencing responsibility grief needs to involve verbal recognition of the individuality of the companion animal; for example, 'Oliver had such a big personality, he was unique. I can understand how you came to be so attached to him'; and acknowledgement of the significance of the relationship, for example, 'Ellie has been with you through so much since you lost your wife, she's helped you through some tough times'.

Caregivers should be given clear, easy-to-understand information about the disease process, both verbal and written, together with opportunities for clarification of information and asking of questions in nurse-facilitated continuing (palliative) care clinics. Clear verbal and written information about, and access to options for, further tests (to confirm diagnosis)/referral and for palliative treatment and care should be given. It is vital not to make assumptions based on value judgements about owners' assumed financial situations; everyone should be given equal access to a range of options and practice/referral services. It is helpful to have an option for home euthanasia, if practical in terms of animal welfare, and to give a sensitive and thorough explanation of the euthanasia process with opportunities for asking questions. It is useful to offer a cognitive reframing of euthanasia as a caring, responsible act within a continuum of a duty of care for our companion animals; for example, 'You've always done everything you can for Hovis and cared for him so well. A last option within palliative care is euthanasia, enabling him to die peacefully without any pain. This is a responsible option even though it's never an easy one'.

Offers of emotional support by familiar veterinary nurses, to enable owners to be present at the time of euthanasia, can be offered simply; for example, 'We've all become fond of Sooty whilst we've been caring for her, I've spent a lot of time with her over the past few weeks and if you would like I could be with you at the time'.

Owners should have enough dedicated time not to have felt rushed in making important decisions, such as choices about further medical investigations, palliative treatments and care options, review of subjective (from owners' perspective) and clinical quality-of-life indicators, euthanasia decision making, deciding about after-death body care, at the time of the euthanasia itself and when collecting ashes from the surgery, and should feel enabled to make the right choice (for themselves) regarding options for after-death body care (home burial, individual cremation, communal/routine cremation and pet cemetery burial). Encouraging rituals for remembrance and enabling continued respect for pets' bodies after death can be powerful in validating grief and making owners feel visible as legitimate grievers mourning the loss of a significant family member.

After death, owners should be supported and encouraged in acceptance of personal responsibility for the euthanasia, with an emphasis that this is a caring act within a continuum of a duty of care for their pet and is grounded in clinical information and advice from the veterinary team responsible for the care of their companion animal. They should be given verbal and written information about grief related to pet loss, including where and how to access pet loss support (such as pet loss support group at the practice, Blue Cross/SCAS PBSS and written details of extended support if needed, for example, Cruse Bereavement Care for issues related to grief arising from human deaths).

Responsibility grief (Dawson 2007a) places specific communication demands on professionals in relation to owners' need for clearly, simply explained clinical information, enabling review of options for treatment and care. Where the veterinary team has not enabled collaborative review of quality-of-life indicators within euthanasia decision making, the likelihood of owners experiencing protracted feelings of doubt and guilt in relation to both the timing and the appropriateness of euthanasia is significantly increased. This may complicate the grieving process and could result in feelings of hostility towards the veterinary surgeon responsible for the care and death of their pet. It may further lead to a reluctance and inability to acquire or even contemplate acquiring a new pet and failure to return to the practice again if a new pet is acquired. Compassionate communication is therefore right at the heart of veterinary practice directly influencing personal experiences of grief, professional responses to management of loss and, ultimately, client loyalty and retention. It makes sound business sense at multiple levels to identify responsibility grief (Dawson 2007a) as being a significant challenge within practice for owners and professionals alike and respond to this positively and proactively.

The unique human needs arising from responsibility grief (Dawson 2007a) can be more adequately met through the introduction of the following:

- Bond-centred practice protocols enabling equality of provision of emotional support
- Ongoing development and review of key skills facilitating compassionate communication, for example active listening
- Provision of nurse-facilitated continuing (palliative) care clinics
- Introduction of illness trajectory mapping as a clinical communication tool
- Enabling access to nurse-facilitated bereavement clinics – functioning as natural extensions of continuing care clinics
- Provision of grief information, details of access to pet bereavement support, for example The Blue Cross/SCAS PBSS

- Attention to environmental and physical resource considerations, for example
  - having a dedicated family/quiet room where stressed and distressed owners can spend time with their companion animals and practice staff
  - sending of condolence cards to bereaved owners
  - having resources to enable making of 'linking items', for example clay paw moulds, paw print making, fur swatch envelopes

These are all crucial resources in communicating genuine compassion and acknowledging the personal significance of the individual person–pet bond.

Pet loss is a contextual loss, which means it does not occur in isolation but within the wider context of people's lives and experiences. Some owners by virtue of their circumstances and life stage may be more vulnerable to the impact of grief. Recognizing *vulnerability factors* is important in supporting owners to access the emotional support they may need.

Vulnerability factors

Professional interactions with owners give just 'a snapshot in time', providing merely a fragment of the wider context in which both attachment and loss to companion animals occur. There are, however, known factors which increase vulnerability to loss:

- Living alone
- Coexisting or multiple losses, for example previous miscarriage/elective abortion and other human deaths
- Long-term physical chronic illness/other additional needs
- Absence of a support network, for example friends, work colleagues and faith community
- Previous/current emotional health difficulties, for example chronic depression
- Not in current employment/recent redundancy
- Homelessness – living on the streets
- Loss due to traumatic circumstances, for example animal abuse as in domestic violence; natural disasters such as floods, mandatory slaughter due to FMD (foot and mouth disease) outbreak
- Witnessing traumatic death, for example abusive death, road traffic or other accident
- Older age groups with histories of multiple loss and sometimes limited support networks
- Where the pet provided main source of friendship, motivation and purpose
- Where the pet functioned as a linking being for owners, i.e. a living connection with a deceased/absent loved one; practice staff may be unaware of this wider significance unless previously told by owners, further highlighting the importance of never judging individual reactions to loss, which are always contextual

Owners may be reminded of past pets and human losses when visiting the surgery, becoming absorbed in their own thoughts or avoidant of particular consult rooms. These are all normal human responses to grief and sensitive management can be worked with to enable owners to be in the here and now of the consult with their present companion animal. Taking a BCVP approach can enable an increased ability to recognize and respond to owners' individual needs. Putting bond-centred principles in place, ensuring protocols for provision of emotional support are agreed and adhered to, can provide greater equality of care for all owners. BCVP enables compassionate communication at multiple levels. It is therefore useful at this point to clarify what BCVP is.

BCVP focuses on relationships:

- of people with their pets, the HCAB;
- between practice team members and pet owners (staff and clients);
- between practice team members and companion animals cared for;
- between each other as practice team members.

Undoubtedly, professional concerns relating to the possibility of accusations of sentimentality, along with a perceived need to retain some clinical detachment, have inadvertently prevented veterinary professionals from facing the less comfortable territory of navigating human emotions. Essentially a bond-centred approach to veterinary practice does exactly this – it involves veterinary professionals recognizing, acknowledging and responding to owners' emotional needs through provision of appropriate emotional support.

A bond-centred practice supports and responds to emotional needs created by the HCAB (Lagoni et al. 2001). Owners' emotional needs can be identified as follows:

- Trust in the veterinary team – gained through honesty, familiarity, a sense of equality generated by involvement in decisions regarding treatment and care.
- Personalized focused attention – a bespoke service, for example enabled through uninterrupted consults, allowing enough time for each consultation, active verbal recognition of the individual pet–person bond.
- Information – from multiple sources, for example practice website, given verbally in consultations; written information in leaflet/handout form; verbal and written in nurse-facilitated clinics.
- Acknowledgement of and response to the HCAB – verbal recognition of the individuality of the companion animal; validation of the relationship between pets and people; active support to maintain the bond, for example through provision of community nursing for housebound owners or those with other additional needs, access to practice-enabled temporary pet fostering at times of crisis.
- Knowledge about animal behaviour, how to solve problems and access to referrals to other competent professionals if needed.
- Confidence in the veterinary team's ability to identify and respond to sensitive issues.
- Validation of intuition, observations and perceptions regarding their pet's health – involving listening to and valuing owners' subjective perspectives, which can be enabled through applied use of illness trajectory mapping (Dawson 2007a).
- Compassionate communication skills to soothe anxiety and fear, resolve conflict and enable exploration of treatment and care options.
- Direct honest communication – for example avoiding the use of confusing euphemisms such as 'put to sleep,' replacing with 'helped to die peacefully'.
- A feeling of partnership during decision making and treatment procedures, enabled through developing *active listening skills*, utilizing clinical communication tools, for example illness trajectory mapping and through provision of a diverse range of nurse-facilitated clinics, for example nutrition and weight management; continuing care (palliative care), dental and behaviour clinics.

- Access to veterinarian/other professional approachable available staff, developing a sense of the surgery as a community resource with an 'open door' policy.
- Skilled, professional, boundaried support (not spilling over into personal friendships, e.g. giving out home telephone numbers, trying to provide counselling about wider issues when not trained, insured or supervised to do so); support during crises – whilst some owners will deal with emotional distress in their own way privately and will decline support offered, a majority will value additional time spent with them in a supportive capacity, for example terminal diagnosis/prognosis, euthanasia decision making, pre-, during and post-euthanasia of their companion animals. It is essential to keep this intervention within clear boundaries, in terms of not befriending clients, but instead offering professional, time-limited, emotional support that recognizes and is governed by limitations and competencies.
- Empathy – trying to see the world 'as if' we were the client ourselves, without losing that 'as if' quality. Empathy can provide a unique window into a client's emotional world, enabling identification of issues that may obstruct a client acting in the best interests of an animal's welfare (adapted from the original guidelines as developed by Lagoni et al. 2001).

Bond-centred practice protocols

Protocols need to be agreed and invested in by the whole team and not imposed by one dominant team member. What is practical, given operational and environmental limitations, needs to be taken into account. Staff training needs should also be identified and addressed to facilitate implementation, alongside attention to basic environmental considerations, such as provision of a quiet area or room for use during crises where owners will not feel rushed or be interrupted.

Particular focus areas for consideration for development of BCVP protocols (see Table 4.2) which enable effective working with human emotions in practice include the following:

- Animal selection, advice on choice of pets before acquisition
- Behaviour management
- Puppy socializing
- Weight management
- Enabling and supporting compliance

Table 4.2 Areas for bond-centred veterinary practice protocols

Client-Centred Guidelines	Staff-Centred Guidelines	Community-Centred Guidelines
Client 'quiet room'/ comfort room	Protocol for delivering terminal prognosis	Hospice care
Handouts	Protocol for staff debriefings	Self-help support groups
Grief information packs		
PBSS details		

- Crisis response, for example temporary fostering of animals for owners
- Responding to suspected non-accidental injury including agencies to be informed, for example social services, Police CPU (Child Protection Unit), and the Royal Society for the Prevention of Cruelty to Animals (RSPCA)
- Palliative treatment and care
- Euthanasia
- Pet loss support
- Staff communication
- Staff support

Each of these areas should essentially accommodate provision of staff emotional support networks, for example, peer support by colleagues, enabling external access to professional counselling if needed. Provision of appropriate training for practice team members should always be included along with identification of environmental and resource implications, enabling effective implementation.

Example: euthanasia emotional support protocols (Dawson 2007a)

To ensure continuity and equality of access to care, putting in place euthanasia protocols can enable practice staff to feel more confident in supporting owners in the time leading up to, the time of, and following, the euthanasia of the companion animal. Suggested issues for inclusion within euthanasia protocols for communication and client care are listed below with a brief explanation of their significance in supporting owners and communicating empathy at what can be a difficult and stressful time:

1. Development of a dedicated quiet/family room or area, enabling owners to spend time with their pets as a family; provision of paper tissues, water/hot drink easily available, comfortable seating, a comfortable area for the pet to lie or sit on (alternatives to consult tables such as soft mats). Generation of a less clinical environment through integration of plants and pictures of animals, attention paid to the colour of the room walls, for example pale blue and pale green are perceived to be colours that calm and sooth emotions.
2. Access to physical resources within the quiet room, for example clay paw moulds, grief education packs, children's books about pet loss.
3. Veterinary teams being prepared for the euthanasia beforehand (where possible), for example communicating why Mrs Jones is bringing Pippa in at the end of surgery to avoid inadvertent creation of the wrong emotional environment or inappropriate/insensitive comments; the veterinary surgeon having prepared the euthanasia syringe out of sight of owners, knowing the weight of the animal beforehand. This communicates sensitivity and respect for the animal and owner. It can also lessen stress for both owners and professionals.
4. Extended appointment time with a veterinary surgeon, or nurse, familiar with the individual animal and disease trajectory, enabling adequate information gathering and time for a physical examination to inform the euthanasia decision making within a personal context. This is essential in facilitating a thorough review of quality-of-life indicators (subjective and clinical) and in confirming the decision to euthanize as being in the interest of the animal's welfare (altruistic motivation). This is very important in lessening

feelings of doubt and guilt, clarifying owners' altruistic motivation and reducing the potential for feelings of hostility and resentment towards the professionals responsible for the euthanasia, an important consideration in client retention when acquiring new pets in the future.

5. Clear explanation and clarification of the euthanasia procedure including possible observed physiological responses of the animal, for example agonal gasp, involuntary urination/defaecation, the eyes remaining open after death; enabling questions which should be answered honestly, avoiding confusing euphemisms such as 'put to sleep,' and instead using more truthful explanations, 'helped to die peacefully without any pain or distress'. This helps to prepare owners and eliminate unpleasant imaginings generated through ignorance. Using honest terms to reinforce the irreversibility and seriousness of the event is helpful in enabling acceptance and essentially generating an understanding of what the procedure results in – the death of the animal.

6. Enough time allowed for euthanasia decision making and for the euthanasia event, for example schedule an end-of-surgery appointment where possible. Can be useful in reducing doubt in relation to the appropriateness and timing of the euthanasia. Enables a sense of dignity for owners and companion animals; communicates respect.

7. An option for home euthanasia by the regular veterinarian responsible for the companion animal without protracted time delay for an appointment where operationally possible and practical in terms of animal welfare. Can be vital to owners' sense of agency, validates family member status of the pet and communicates respect for the individuality of the relationship and needs arising from this.

8. Ensuring familiarity of the veterinarian or nurse present with the companion animal (where feasibly possible), very significant in personalization of the procedure, recognition of the individuality of the companion animal.

9. Pre-euthanasia examination of the animal validating the euthanasia decision. This is essential in confirming there are no current alternative options available other than euthanasia (if this is truthfully the case). Can lessen feelings of doubt and associated guilt.

10. Owners not being required to be active agents in the process of euthanasia, for example assisting in raising a vein as this can be traumatic, magnifying owners' sense of personal responsibility and guilt associated with euthanasia.

11. Having an option of physically comforting an animal during the euthanasia procedure, for example owners holding their animal's head to provide comfort and lessen distress; integral in recognizing the family status of most pets, enabling a sense of maintained trust and continued care. This passive involvement can increase owners' sense of agency within the euthanasia process, whilst not actively involving them in the procedure itself.

12. Active confirmation of death in front of owners – involving the veterinary surgeon visibly listening for a heartbeat with a stethoscope and verbally confirming death. This was revealed as being fundamental in helping acceptance of the reality of the loss and pivotal in slowing down the rapid flux of the dynamic dialectic of responsibility grief, enabling a shift from anticipation to actualization of feelings.

13. After-death continued care – arranging the pet's body in a sleeping position, cleaning up any urine or faeces, closing the eyes. Refraining from putting the pet into a clinical waste bag in front of owners and, where the owners are taking the body home for disposal, having blankets available for discrete and sensitive removal. If polythene

sheets/body bags are needed due to body fluid leakage, sensitive explanation should be given to owners of why this is advisable. If veterinary team members treat deceased companion animals' bodies with continued care and respect at all times, this communicates integrity, genuineness, compassion and care towards both companion animals and owners. It further validates the significance of the individual companion animal and the status of owners as legitimate grievers worthy of treatment with respect and dignity.

14. Enabling owners to spend time post-death with their companion animal, ideally through provision of a 'quiet room' to compose self and spend time with their deceased animal before leaving the practice, which should ideally be via a separate exit not involving them walking through the waiting room.

15. With the owner's permission, creating linking items for remembrance – this involves cutting a swatch of fur (which should be given to owners sensitively in a small dedicated plastic bag – not a biohazard bag), making a paw print for owners to keep or a clay paw mould (see Figure 4.2). Helps to create rituals for remembrance, validates the loss as significant and communicates respect for the pet's individuality.

16. Sensitive explanation of options for after-death body disposal, such as cremation, including information about alternatives (e.g. home or pet cemetery burial). This is essential in enabling rituals of remembrance and active respect for the companion animal.

17. Giving verbal acknowledgement of the personal significance of the individual companion animal, the bond between the owner and the animal, and the significance of the impact of the death. Integral within the dynamic of responsibility grief is the

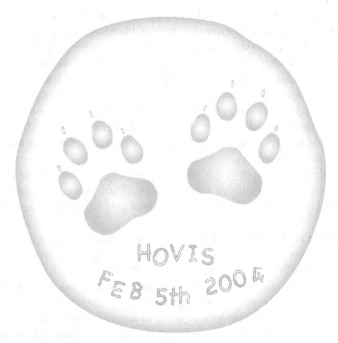

Figure 4.2 Clay paw mould.

disenfranchisement of this loss. In having their grief validated this helps put a name to the uncomfortable feelings experienced and normalizes them as acceptable within this context.

18. Written provision of grief education – can be helpful in legitimization of feelings, particularly uncomfortable feelings such as guilt, egoism, selfishness and doubt. Enables recognition and naming of emotions, alongside practical information about accessing extended support, for example through in-practice bereavement clinics or via The Blue Cross/SCAS PBSS.

19. Provision of a back door exit to leave the surgery to avoid walking through the waiting room. Important in communicating recognition of the significance of the loss and of the caregiver as a griever, worthy of sensitive and dignified treatment.

20. Not having to pay the veterinary bill at the time of euthanasia as a request for payment can be perceived as insensitive; alternatively, taking payment over the telephone at the time of booking the euthanasia appointment, before the event or sending the bill (to known clients) a few days afterwards can be more thoughtful ways of settling associated financial transactions.

21. Providing the option of talking through feelings and memories with a nurse who knew the animal personally at the time of collecting the ashes from the veterinary surgery, rather than picking these up from the reception desk, which could be perceived as impersonal and objectifying. This could be a vital function of a practice bereavement clinic. This can enable validation of both the relationship and the loss as significant, rather than inconsequential or routine. It importantly creates a lasting positive memory and association with the practice, enabling return if another animal is acquired, or for the treatment of remaining pets.

22. Sending out a personalized bereavement card from the practice, written by the attending members of the team who knew the animal. Handwriting should always be legible; the card ideally should depict a tranquil scene (avoiding the potential for offence if animals are pictured, which may not be the right breed or type, as this could cause further distress or offence for owners) and should be sent 2–3 days after the death. A packet of forget-me-not seeds for planting in remembrance can be an excellent, subtle way of communicating care, which encourages rituals of remembrance for companion animals. Bills for euthanasia should *never* be sent out with bereavement cards. Avoid religious-oriented cards to respect the diversity of different faiths of owners and those who do not hold any religious beliefs.

23. Provision of time-limited pet bereavement support by the practice, for example pet loss support groups, nurse-facilitated bereavement clinics. Basic provision should ideally consist of grief information and referral details of how to contact The Blue Cross/SCAS PBSS.

24. Each consulting room and reception should carry contact details and information on referral agencies for pet loss support and extended support. Team members should enable clients to have the option of contacting the PBSS for immediate pet loss support. In more critical situations, where a client expresses a need for wider support, staff should feel confident in verbally recommending a client to seek referral from their general practitioner to a primary care counsellor or other professional qualified to work with wider presenting issues of a more serious and urgent nature, for example in relation to human bereavements and/or other coexisting emotional health issues.

25.   Vulnerable clients perceived to be at risk should be offered the option of a member of the practice team contacting a family member or other carer who could be with them after the death. Alternatively, in some circumstances, with the client's permission, referral to social services by the practice may be appropriate. Written and verbal details of how to contact the Samaritans should also be provided for clients experiencing more extensive emotional health issues (adapted from Dawson 2007a, pp. 477–480).

Protocols should include explicit identification of where staff can elicit and access support for themselves, both within and outside the practice, for example, from a named member of the practice team, Vetlife website, referral via employee assistance for dedicated external support. It should never be assumed that being in the presence of the intense emotions of others on a daily basis and having professional responsibility for ending life do not impact in some way on everyone in practice. Just as with clients, professionals do not live in a vacuum but experience these stresses in the context of other events happening at home. Team members may not be consciously aware of the emotional impact of repeated exposure to owners' distress or responsibility for euthanasia is having on them, but this does not mean that the impact is any less real or serious. Communicating clearly about what support is available and how this can be accessed is important within BCVP as a fundamental of developing and sustaining positive relationships between team members that naturally extends to provision of cohesive approaches to client care.

Staff emotional support sessions are a useful tool to facilitate open communication amongst team members about the emotional consequences of working with human grief and other emotions on a daily basis. These should be facilitated by someone who is able to manage the session, enabling everyone who wants to have say, to do so and sum up emerging themes and patterns, clarifying any action points. These could be integrated before regular staff team meetings, but should not be optional, as ideally, most of the staff team should attend. A weekly staff emotional support session will help to:

- develop a culture of safety and care for team members, as well as clients, based on keeping communication channels open;
- negotiate agendas, reduce uncertainty about change and implement/evaluate emotional support protocols;
- build a supportive environment for open discussion and sharing of feelings, essentially extending the emotion-friendly environment created for owners to staff;
- motivate whole practice participation in emotional support for owners and for each other, fostering a sense of collective responsibility;
- share information;
- resolve conflict and feelings of anger in a secure environment;
- encourage staff to accept feedback and reflect on the practice of emotional support provision.

Acknowledging and working with both the emotions of owners and veterinary team members contribute towards the creation of a culture of care and an emotion-friendly environment. Central within this is compassionate communication, which enables veterinary professionals to retain personal composure and maintain a professional distance, whilst simultaneously being empathic and communicating this to clients.

Compassionate communication skills

Burnard and Morrison (1997) reflect that caring and communicating are inseparably linked. Clear, respectful communication is as vital to the success of bond-centred practice as high-quality medical care. Trust is the foundation of effective communication and of healthy work environments. 'A bond-centred practice creates work environments characterized by high levels of trust and skilled communication' (Lagoni et al. 2001).

Compassion tends to be action-focused, associated with sympathy and help. Thompson (1986), writing about communication in health care, posits that communication is important for two main reasons: it facilitates the sharing of information and it enables relationships between people.

Communication is thus a two-way process. There are different types of communication that can be used to convey compassion and offer support.

Oral communication involves using words and sentences (verbal communication); for example, 'I think I know how much Fennel meant to you, Zoe; please take all the time you need now, there's no rush to leave'. Body language (non-verbal communication) involves, for example, a relaxed open posture and the use of eye contact. Written communication involves sending a personalized sympathy card, for example.

There are key skills and orientations involved in communicating compassionately and these are now introduced and discussed with examples related to veterinary practice.

Empathy

This is more a way of being, an orientation rather than a skill, that can be learned and practiced. Egan (1986) defines empathy as being the ability to enter into and understand the world of another person and communicate this understanding to him or her. The crucial factor is retaining an 'as if' quality. In this way empathy is different to sympathy. Empathy involves both an intellectual and emotional understanding of the other person's experience. Egan (1986), however, also identifies empathy as being a communication skill, that of accurately communicating understanding of the emotions and thoughts of another. In this way, the skill of empathizing with another's experience is grounded in *active listening*.

Active listening

Listening is different to hearing; we can hear sounds without making sense of them. Listening involves giving full attention in an effort to understand what is being said, verbally and non-verbally. For more information on listening, please see Chapter 1. Veterinary professionals' active listening involves communicating this understanding to companion animal owners effectively, both verbally and non-verbally, through the following:

- Tone of voice and pace of speech – for example, mirroring owners' pace of speech can also communicate empathy.
- Eye contact.
- Attending – involves communicating to someone that you are paying close attention to what is being said and expressed, for example use of relaxed, open body language.

- Clarifying – a central skill in communicating care is building understanding by checking out what the person has said. This can be done through paraphrasing, restating and the use of open questions.
- Probes and prompts – a probe is an exploratory question; for example, 'Can you tell me more about what is worrying you about Angel's cancer?' This type of question usually follows on from a previous answer given; for example, 'I'm just worried about the cancer.' Prompts are short questions or words which you offer to someone in order to prompt an answer; for example, 'Does Angel seem distressed?' Be aware, however, that it is better to avoid such leading questions outside end-of-life discussions.
- Summarizing.

There are extremely emotionally charged times in practice, however, as illustrated in Case Study 4.1, that challenge professionals' active listening and demand a need for further expansive compassionate communication skills.

Case Study 4.1 Baby

Baby was an 8-year-old female Staffordshire bull terrier that was dead on arrival at the out-of-hours emergency hospital, as a result of multiple injuries sustained in an RTA (road traffic accident). Sandy had owned Baby since she was 3 years old, when she adopted her from an RSPCA animal centre. Sandy is 32 years old and has three children, Kylie aged 4 years, Bethany aged 7 years and George who is 10 years old. George was holding Baby's lead at the time she slipped her collar just before the accident and blames himself for her death. Sandy, whilst distraught at Baby's loss, did not seem to blame George. However, Liam (Sandy's partner and George's father), was extremely angry towards George and towards the practice team for 'letting Baby die'. He was shouting uncontrollably at George, swearing at the vet and nurse, who found it impossible to calm him down. Other people in the waiting room were also becoming anxious and distressed because they could hear what was going on.

The whole family accompanied Baby to the surgery and the consulting room was very crowded. The vet and nurse were eager to get Liam out of the hospital. Sandy appeared numb and in a state of shock. The vet explained that Baby had died before she had arrived at the hospital and emphasized that nothing could be done now to help her. The nurse was concerned to watch that Kylie and Bethany did not touch anything in the room as the girls were actively exploring this new environment and seemed unaware that Baby was dead.

The family were not provided with the information regarding individual cremation and left Baby's body at the hospital for communal cremation, which Sandy later deeply regretted.

This case study highlights diverse factors that can impact on human grief in relation to pet loss:

- Sudden, unanticipated death of a younger animal
- Possible existence of responsibility/culpability for the death

- Traumatic death, for example accident
- Unfamiliar veterinary team, presenting issues of questioning trust in competency
- Rescued animal
- Discrepant (different) grieving styles within family systems

The emotional climate is highly charged, presenting multiple layers of differing needs. Liam's anger is a natural part of grief, particularly in relation to accidental death. Sandy's shock and disbelief is making it easy to overlook Sandy, as all the attention may have inadvertently been focused on calming Liam down. The children in the family present different levels of understanding about death and dying; Kylie and Bethany appear not to understand the gravity of the situation and need simple explanation to help them realize what had happened to Baby. George, as a child, is taking the full burden of responsibility for Baby's death, which he understands was preventable and is a permanent state, and this is further complicated by Liam's anger towards George.

The veterinary team do not know the family personally and therefore do not have a foundation of trust and familiarity to work from. It becomes essential to manage this traumatic loss situation compassionately and calmly for the family by the following:

- Identifying immediate priorities for concern – diffusing Liam's anger by remaining gently spoken when talking to Liam, advising him, that feelings of anger are a natural part of grief particularly in relation to accidental death.
- Allowing Liam a few minutes to externalize his feelings without interrupting him and not becoming angry in response.
- The vet further clarifying that it is normal, but not helpful to want to blame someone for accidental death.
- Offering to explain Baby's injuries that led to her death in front of the family and doing so when the environment becomes more stable and focussed to enable greater understanding.
- Ensuring that Sandy and Liam have somewhere to sit down.
- Providing the option for involvement of the children or alternatively offering a member of staff who could talk to the children in a separate room about the loss, whilst the vet works with Sandy and Liam.

Missing My Pet by Alex Lambert (aged 6) is an extremely helpful resource for explaining death to children in practice and could be used by the nurse with the children; ideally, the book should be available to give to the family before they go home, included within the grief information pack. The book has an accompanying parent/carers' pamphlet, which provides down-to-earth guidance on explaining pet death to children. Use age-appropriate language with the children, avoiding euphemisms such as 'gone to sleep/passed away,' instead use the words 'dead' and 'died', clarifying that this means that Baby's heart has stopped beating, she has stopped breathing, she does not feel pain and she is not frightened.

The family as a whole, including the children, should be allowed to say their goodbyes to Baby, touch her if they would like to (helpful in accepting the reality of the loss), make a paw print/clay paw mould to help remember her and generate an opportunity for ritual (enabling expression/externalization of feelings).

Ideally, the family should be able to decide together about options regarding after-death body care, and should be provided with different alternatives for this; decisions could be made the next day. It is important *not* to rush the family, who are struggling to come to terms with Baby's sudden death, or to make assumptions about the family's financial circumstances and possible limitations.

It is essential that the veterinary care team involved in working with the family are provided with an opportunity to take a few minutes to collect their own thoughts before working with new clients, if possible. Opportunities for staff to debrief with an identified team member should be ensured at the end of each shift; this may be face to face or by telephone.

Further compassionate communication skills that can help generate a more emotion-friendly environment, typical of a bond-centred practice, include the following:

- Acknowledging – recognizing the existence of personal truth or the reality of a situation for another person. It involves observational comments and statements about the bond between owners and their pets as well as honest communication about stressful and emotionally difficult subjects such as delivering a terminal prognosis, and reflecting on the human emotions associated with grief and loss; for example, 'Baby's death has come as a massive shock to all of you and it looks like everyone in the family is trying to cope with this in their own way'.
- Normalizing – this lends credibility to another's thoughts, beliefs, behaviours and experiences and enables owners to know that their reactions are 'normal'. It involves offering validation to owners about the emotions associated with grief and other stressful situations such as euthanasia, 'Feelings of anger and wanting to blame someone are a natural part of grief, particularly in association with accidental death'.
- Giving permission – encouraging owners to articulate their needs and wishes without anxiety and without feeling judged. Owners perceive and relate to veterinary professionals as authority figures, sometimes owners need to have permission to be able to make choices regarding their pets' welfare and care such as ending treatment or reviewing quality-of-life indicators; Sandy may need permission to grieve; for example, 'Would you like to spend some time alone with Baby? It's OK to do this if you need to, and we can make a print of her paw if you'd like this …'.
- Gentle confrontation, 'Baby slipped her collar, this wasn't anyone's fault and nobody is to blame, it is likely she died at the scene of the accident. There was nothing we could do for her when she arrived'.
- Immediacy, 'Would it help if Lisa took the children next door for a few moments whilst you and your wife spend some time with Baby and the vet?'

Natural human reactions to working with Baby's family could include frustration, irritation and avoidance. In remaining calm and mirroring what is the desired way of being, the veterinary team generate a climate that can lessen conflict, rather than exacerbate it. Empathy enables understanding of the source of Liam's anger that, whilst difficult to work in the presence of, is based in shock, distress and grief. In focusing on working with the *person* and their emergent needs rather than responding to the emotions, professionals are better able to deflect anger and avoid it escalating into aggression.

Case Study 4.2 illustrates how compassionate communication skills can enable an emotionally supported transition for owners at the time of terminal prognosis and euthanasia of their companion animal.

Case Study 4.2 Willow

Bill purchased Willow (a Siamese cat) from a breeder as a present for his wife's birthday, 10 years ago. He describes Willow as being 'the most beautiful kitten' he had ever seen and talks of her becoming 'his cat', although he had initially bought her for his wife. Bill and his wife, Mary, live in a rural area of Cheshire and have two grown-up children who live overseas. Bill is a retired university lecturer, in his late 60s. Mary, also in her late 60s, has multiple sclerosis (MS) and uses a wheelchair. Bill describes Willow as being friendly, very communicative and sociable. She was 10 years old when she was euthanized at home due to skin cancer. Willow was diagnosed over a year before she eventually died. When the lesion first appeared on Willow's nose, Bill hadn't thought it was serious, but when he finally went to see his vet, Willow was diagnosed as having a malignancy and the vet operated to remove this. The vet provided straightforward information about Willow's cancer, describing the anticipated trajectory. He did not assume that because Bill was a university lecturer he would automatically understand medical terminology. Bill was interested in learning as much as possible about what he could do to support Willow during her palliative treatment and care. He was advised to attend a continuing care (palliative) clinic at the surgery. This is facilitated by a qualified nurse, fully trained in provision of pet bereavement support. He attended four appointments (one per month after prognosis), each lasting around 20 minutes. During the consultations Bill was able to talk about his relationship with Willow, explore his fears and anxieties about Willow's cancer, identify practical steps he could take to ensure Willow's comfort, locate and explore key quality-of-life indicators (Willow's mobility, the appearance and size of the tumour, appetite and zest for life), access information about euthanasia and options of where this could eventually take place. Bill had talked with Mary and they had decided that Willow would be buried at home in the garden, where she enjoyed playing; consequently, they did not require details of cremation or pet cemetery services. The nurse advised Bill that Willow's grave would need to be dug to a depth of 1.25 m, as this was a legal requirement, but she also commented that home burial seemed an appropriate choice for Willow, as she enjoyed being out in the garden so much.

Willow, despite her terminal prognosis, recovered from surgery and had 'a good summer,' but as winter approached she got rapidly worse. She was losing weight, the tumour returned and visibly bled; Bill talked of it being 'obvious' by May of the following year that 'she was not herself anymore.' Willow had 3 weeks in a 'fairly low state', and eventually got so she was not moving around and the tumour had caused considerable facial disfigurement. Bill identified that Willow was in discomfort. Willow's familiar vet and the continuing (palliative) care nurse came to Bill's home to euthanize Willow. The vet examined Willow thoroughly, talking Bill and Mary through this examination, verbally validating the reasons for the euthanasia decision. The vet explained the euthanasia procedure to them, identifying aspects which may have caused distress or alarm, for example, the possibility that Willow's bowels and bladder may empty, that her eyes would remain open after death and that she may sound as if she was sighing or gasping, clarifying that this is a reflex after death and not a sign that she was in distress. After allowing an opportunity for questions, the vet briefly outlined what the euthanasia consent form was and why it was needed, before asking Bill to complete it. Mary felt she couldn't stay in the room at the time of the euthanasia, but Bill remained and stroked Willow whilst the vet injected her. Bill was not required to raise a vein. The procedure went peacefully and Bill said he was in no doubt that it was the appropriate choice for Willow at this stage to prevent her from suffering. Mary was invited back into the room. The vet acknowledged that he would miss Willow, as she had a big personality and was such a sociable cat. The continuing care nurse provided Bill and Mary with written contact details of where he could access pet bereavement support should he need it, ensuring he had contact details for Blue Cross/SCAS PBSS. The vet and attending nurse sent a handwritten bereavement card to the couple, from the practice, the next day. The invoice for euthanasia was sent 1 week after Willow's death. Neither Bill nor his wife pursued the option of external bereavement support, but talked of appreciating having the information, which gave them a choice. Bill commented that he felt the practice had been compassionate and very genuine in relation to Willow's illness and eventual death.

It could have been easy for Willow's vet to make assumptions about what Bill, as a university lecturer, might want and need in terms of information and potential pet bereavement support. It could also have been easy to have excluded Mary from the euthanasia, had there not been an option for home visits, as the practice did not have easy access for people who use wheelchairs. Despite the fact Mary felt she could not remain in the room at the time of death, she was able to participate in the part of the process she felt more comfortable with, enabling validation of the euthanasia decision and clarification of the appropriateness of its timing. In the practice, being committed to equality of access and continuity of care, the vet and the nurse were able to respond more flexibly to owners' individual needs. The practice team worked with Bill (and also with Mary when able to do so) in a person-centred way from their frame of reference, using empathy and enabling recognition of Mary and Bill as individuals with different ways of coping with anticipatory grief and at the time of Willow's euthanasia. Compassionate communication and practical support were enabled by the vet and nurse following collaboratively agreed practice protocols for provision of palliative and bereavement care. Key areas of importance within this included the following:

- Verbal recognition of the HCAB (validating the relationship)
- Acknowledgement of the individuality and significance of the companion animal
- Provision of clear, easily understood information regarding the disease trajectory, enabling Willow's owners to identify what role they could take in her continuing care (owner empowerment)
- An option for home euthanasia, if preferred
- Pre-euthanasia examination of Willow, followed by discussion of quality-of-life indicators, making visible the reason for the euthanasia and its timing, lessening the potential for doubt and associated feelings of guilt (locating altruistic motivation for the death)
- Providing details of how and where to access support should it have been needed
- Pet bereavement is always contextual, i.e. happens within the wider context of people's lives; it is therefore helpful to be aware of potential vulnerability factors, for example:

○ Coexisting multiple losses experienced by Bill and Mary, for example Bill's re-tirement, Mary's MS and subsequent loss of mobility. Extended support may be needed from other agencies such as social services, MS Society, Age Concern.

○ Access to support networks/structures, for example family members. Both of Bill and Mary's children live overseas; therefore, it could be useful to check out if they have contact with other family members, friends, faith/social groups they can eas-ily access.

○ Intensity of the HCAB within owner dyads, for example Bill's identification that Willow was 'his cat', illuminating the special bond he perceived they shared.

○ Older age-related factors, for example emergent anxiety in owners relating to their own mortality brought into consciousness as a result of pet bereavement.

○ 'Last pet syndrome', older people sometimes feel they cannot responsibly assume a caring commitment for another animal because of fear that they may outlive the pet, gentle reassurance of home for life schemes with details of these can be helpful if owners want to have another companion animal; providing written information about the Cinnamon Trust (pet fostering and rehoming charity for elderly pet own-ers) may be crucial in enabling future acquisition of a new pet. Owners can also be advised of older animals in need of new homes.

○ Guilt associated with aspects of the caring responsibility, for example Bill may have felt guilty for not having taken Willow to see the vet sooner, as by the time of diagnosis the cancer had already spread; Mary may also feel guilty she felt unable to remain with Willow at the time of her death.

Supportive actions taken by the practice care team that were useful in working with the human emotions associated with these vulnerability factors included the following:

• Clear, compassionate communication – honesty from the start regarding the termi-nal prognosis, informing Bill that the tumour was malignant, making it clear that the surgery was palliative and not curative; explanation of the suspected illness trajectory, clear description of euthanasia procedure with opportunities for questions.

• Access to continuing (palliative) care clinics at the practice, enabling more expansive discussion, review of the pet–person relationship, locating important factors within quality of life and empowerment of Bill within the palliative care process for Willow, enabling him to identify options and clarify his own role as Willow's primary care-giver.

• An option for home-based euthanasia by the regular, familiar practice care team, which gave Mary the option to be present at the time of Willow's death.

• Communicating respect and a non-judgemental attitude, in acceptance of Mary choos-ing not to be present during euthanasia and in relation to the timing of Bill bringing Willow for initial investigations.

• Pre-euthanasia examination of Willow and discussion/review of quality-of-life indi-cators informing the euthanasia decision, validation of this from a clinical perspective, illuminating shared responsibility for Willow's death between the owner and the vet-erinary care team, essential in lessening feelings of doubt in relation to the appropri-ateness of the timing of the euthanasia and subsequent feelings of guilt.

- Information about where to access pet bereavement support if needed – enabling choice, but respecting how owners choose to grieve and what support they decide they need to access.

This case study highlights the importance of both generic procedures and individual responses when working with human emotions associated with palliative care and bereavement in practice. Whilst it is essential to have emotional support protocols that ensure minimum provision of information and access to extended support, it is also necessary to work in a person-centred way, using empathy to identify the more personal needs arising from individual contexts and particular loss circumstances.

REVIEW OF QUALITY-OF-LIFE INDICATORS

In addition to developing compassionate communication skills, there are some potentially useful clinical communication tools that enable more empathic person-centred approaches to working with human emotions relating to reviewing quality-of-life indicators within euthanasia decision making and palliative treatment and care. Essentially, these tools generate a sense of real partnership between owners and professionals. Illness trajectory, or 'bond mapping', can be used at any stage of veterinary treatment and care, but is particularly relevant to palliative and bereavement care. Illness trajectory mapping, developed by Dawson (2007a), has also been successfully integrated into companion animal bereavement counselling as a means of making visible the factors that influenced and informed euthanasia decision making (see Figure 4.3). The purpose of illness trajectory mapping is:

- to identify personally important facets of the HCAB (located as the roots of the map);
- to locate key moments within the illness trajectory, for example owners' first awareness of disease process/terminal decline, veterinary diagnosis/prognosis, subjective and clinical quality-of-life indicators;
- to identify the pivotal moment, i.e. informing/deciding factor for the euthanasia – which could be generated by a number of key moments or be a discrete event, for example sudden onset of paralysis;
- to make visible the limitations, both in terms of clinical treatment and personal circumstances. For example, is someone at home on a daily basis to care for a terminally ill animal and can the financial costs associated with palliative treatment be managed?

The map also enables identification of factors which help limit feelings of doubt, such as veterinary validation of euthanasia decision, or confirmation of terminal prognosis. Options for euthanasia are highlighted, including involvement of any significant others, such as family members. Owners' personal responsibility for the care and welfare and ultimately the euthanasia of their companion animal is made visible at each step of the mapping process when appropriate.

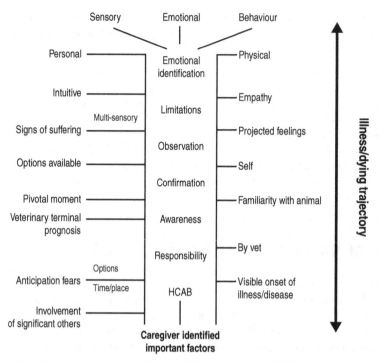

Figure 4.3 Template: illness trajectory mapping (Dawson 2007a).

Professionals' responsibility for the clinical care ensuring animal welfare, clinical information informing euthanasia decision making and, ultimately, for the euthanasia event is made visible, constructing a sense of continued partnership between owners and the veterinary care team.

The map is not considered to be a clinical record nor a crude decision-making tool, but rather a personal review process facilitated by a professional usually working within a continuing (palliative) care clinic.

Owners can be given a photocopy of the map with written information on it, or alternatively the template can be used as a way of identifying verbal discussion areas. It is useful to integrate a written component if possible and appropriate, as this can be valuable for owners to review following the death, revisiting the circumstances informing the decision making. It should always be emphasized, preferably in writing on the template, that this is not a clinical record of euthanasia decision making, but represents a personal process review.

At times of crisis, owners can become confused, panicked or fearful and avoidant of situations that may cause anxiety and further stress, for example reviewing quality-of-life indicators. It can be useful to put into place a structured option to enable owners to face these situations with support. Offering continuing (palliative) care clinics, facilitated by a dedicated qualified nurse, can provide structured opportunities, enabling illness trajectory mapping and form an empathic bridge, supporting transitions throughout the different stages of palliative treatment and care.

Table 4.3   The purpose of continuing (palliative care) clinics

Review HCAB	What is quality of life?
Identify key factors influencing decision	Identify subjective factors
Provide an opportunity for information seeking related to illness	Are there physical, emotional, financial, timing limitations?
Options for euthanasia, chance to enable understanding of procedure	Dignity – does the animal still have dignity?
Explore fears/anxieties about euthanasia	Enabling a supported presence
After-death body care options	Memorialization of the animal

SETTING UP AND RUNNING CONTINUING CARE CLINICS

The purpose of a continuing (palliative) care clinic (see Table 4.3) is to create a supported space in which owners can talk for a longer duration with a continuing care nurse about all aspects of palliative care, including more subjective experiences integral within the HCAB, which may help illuminate companion animals' quality of life. This *partnership in practice* is aimed at empowering owners of terminally ill animals to take an active role in their continued care through enabling access to information, referrals and practical advice, for example possible, suitable food for terminally ill pets.

Access should be open from the time of terminal diagnosis/prognosis, and this should be enabled by an introduction to the dedicated nurse by the vet responsible for the companion animal's care. Posters in practice can also advertise clinic times, in an owner-friendly way (focusing on practical information and advice available and not on euthanasia and death of the animal). The practice may want to produce a dedicated leaflet outlining the purpose and times of continuing care clinics. Appointment times should be longer, allowing 15–20 minutes for each. Ideally, space permitting, a dedicated quiet/family room should be used for these consults. This should be made to look less clinical by adding framed pictures of companion animals, include an area to make hot drinks, have tissues to hand and have comfortable seating. If a separate room is not available, simple measures can be taken to add greater comfort for owners and animals in existing consulting rooms.

Access to continuing care clinics does not end at the time of the companion animal's death, but naturally extends beyond this to provision of pet bereavement support, embracing the concept of continuing care for the owner. It is essential to keep offers of pet bereavement support within boundaries, ensuring that owners are aware that the appointment time is for 20 minutes and that what is being offered is support and not counselling. Professional counsellors have been trained to work with human emotions in a therapeutic context; they are insured and supervised to work in this way. Veterinary professionals are not trained counsellors and have not entered into a contract for working as counsellors with veterinary clients. Pet bereavement support should involve the following:

- Practical advice about after-death body care, individual or routine (communal) cremation, home and pet cemetery burial.
- Grief education.
- Provision of details about how to contact the PBSS.

- Details of local qualified counsellors willing and able to work with pet bereavement, check out the BACP (British Association for Counselling and Psychotherapy) website for details.
- Contact information relating to other loss issues, for example Cruse Bereavement Care (human losses).
- Memorializing of companion animals, for example adding pets' names to the practice Book of Remembrance, ideas for making a memory box.
- Review of the bond shared with a companion animal.
- Review of end-of-life care, enabling visibility of owners' positive actions.
- Review of euthanasia decision making, enabling identification of altruistic (other-centred) motivation for this (if present) and locating the key and pivotal moments, informing the timing of the euthanasia.
- Information about local or on-site pet bereavement support groups.
- Offering between 2–3 sessions, pet bereavement support helps to ensure that this provision remains within boundaries. Pet bereavement support will not be wanted, nor indeed needed, for a number of owners. It is important not to make assumptions, but to enable access without forcing these options onto owners. One of the most appropriate times for offering this type of appointment could be at the time of picking up pets' ashes from the surgery, rather than doing this at reception in front of a waiting room full of people. It could be more appropriate to allow a longer time duration, adding of the pet's name to the Book of Remembrance and giving owners an option of talking about the pet and/or the loss if needed. Similarly, if available, details of local or practice pet bereavement support groups could be given at this time, reinforcing a positive link with the practice, rather than the more negative memory of the euthanasia appointment.

PET LOSS SUPPORT GROUPS

Support groups are centred in enabling self-help. Facilitated by a professional, individuals are supported to share their experiences and listen to the experiences of others, drawing inner strength from connecting with people who have shared similar crises and situations, and learning about possible coping strategies that others have successfully employed.

The practicalities

Running a pet loss support group requires a quiet space to hold meetings, for example, the reception area when the centre is closed, or more ideally a different room such as an on-site meeting room. It is important that the group is not seen or disturbed. Tissues should be at hand, as should refreshments.

Facilitator

This is a sensitive, demanding role that requires appropriate communication skills, enabling everyone who wants to have a say to do so. It can be useful to have basic counselling skills training, to enable emotional containment and reflecting back to the group what have been the core themes of the meeting, identifying coping strategies that individuals have found helpful.

Timing

A meeting for an hour once every 2–3 weeks is probably the most sustainable option. Whilst a time limit cannot be placed on grief, it can be helpful to have referral contacts at hand and include the reinforcement at the opening of each session that the group is designed not as a social group, but as a support group to help people through a crisis point in their lives. It is important to be clear about what the group is and what it is not.

Vicarious traumatization

While listening to other people's stories of loss and emotional pain, it is possible to feel worse rather than better. The traumatic experience of others may be internalized as the self's experience, which can be unhelpful or even damaging. It is advisable to think very carefully about the practicalities of setting up and running a pet loss support group on-site, not least because of the emotional demands this places on the staff responsible for facilitating the group. Pet loss support groups, if run well, can provide a positive, continued association with the practice and can support owners, enabling them to consider pet ownership again.

Working with human emotions in practice can be personally draining and professionally demanding and requires that staff have adequate and ongoing training and support to avoid burnout and stress.

CPD OPPORTUNITIES

The Blue Cross/SCAS provides a range of pet bereavement support training programmes, evening continuing professional development (CPD) sessions, daylong and distance learning programmes (externally accredited by the Open College Network).

Blue Cross/SCAS Pet Bereavement Support Service
www.scas.org.uk – telephone 01993 825539

RESOURCES AND USEFUL WEBSITES

Blue Cross/SCAS PBSS provides a confidential support line for pet owners and professionals relating to all aspects of pet loss, staffed by trained support volunteers (8.30 am–8.30 pm). Support line 0800 096 6606 (for adults, children and young people)
Online pet memorials – www.bluecross.org.uk
   Email support pbssmail@bluecross.org.uk
   Information, advice and training on all aspects of pet loss and pet loss support
      pbsstraining@bluecross.org.uk
The British Association for Counselling and Psychotherapy – www.bacp.co.uk

Childline – confidential helpline for children to call enabling access to telephone counselling www.childline.org.uk – telephone 0800 1111

Cinnamon Trust (national charity for the elderly and their pets) – www.cinnamontrust.org.uk

Cruse Bereavement Care counselling, advice and support related to *human* deaths only, does not offer pet loss support. Useful in supporting owners who are experiencing multiple losses and requires more extensive support in relation to human bereavement. www.crusebereavementcare.org.uk

   Helpline (9.30 am–5.00 pm) 0808 808 1677

Young People's Helpline 0844 477 9400

Family-friendly grief resources for use in practice, *Missing My Pet* by Alex Lambert (aged 6) with accompanying parent/carers' pamphlet

RSPCA Home for Life – www.homeforlife.org.uk

The Missing Pets Bureau – www.petsbureau.co.uk

Understanding and working with responsibility grief for companion animal owners and professionals – www.responsbilitygrief.co.uk

Vetlife website support for veterinary professionals – www.vetlife.org.uk

REFERENCES

American Veterinary Medical Association (AVMA) (2006) JAVMA news: board acts on human-animal bond issues. *Journal of the American Veterinary Medical Association* 228(2):167–194.

Barton Ross C, Baron-Sorensen J (2007) *Pet Loss and Human Emotions: A Guide to Recovery*, 2nd edn. Routledge, New York.

Beetz AM (2007) The development of empathy in children through interaction with animals. Plenary paper, IAHAIO Conference: People and Animals: Partnership in Harmony, Tokyo.

Bowlby J (1969) *Attachment*. Basic Books, New York.

Bowlby J (1979) *The Making and Breaking of Affectional Bonds*. Tavistock Publications, London.

Bowlby J (1980) *Loss*. Basic Books, New York, p. 93.

Bowlby J (1988) *Secure Base*. Basic Books, New York.

Brown SE (2004a) The human–animal bond and self psychology: toward a new understanding. *Society and Animals, Journal of Human–Animal Studies* 12(1):67–86.

Brown SE (2004b) The human–animal bond: self psychology offers special insight. *PSYETA (Psychologists for the Ethical Treatment of Animals) News* 24(1):4.

Burnard P, Morrison P (1997) *Caring and Communicating: Interpersonal Relationships in Nursing*. Palgrave, Basingstoke, UK.

Cohen SP (2002) Can pets function as family members? *Western Journal of Nursing Research* 26(6):621–638.

Crawford EK, Worsham NL, Swinehart ER (2006) Benefits derived from companion animals and the use of the term 'attachment.' *Anthrozoos* 19(2):98–112.

Dawson SE, Campbell W (2005) Companion animal loss: understanding and supporting older people. In: Dono J, Ormerod E (eds), *Older People and Pets*. SCAS, Oxford, pp. 152–153.

Dawson SE (2006) A disenfranchised loss, companion animal death. *Funeral Services Journal* 121:96–103.

Dawson SE (2007a) Companion animal euthanasia: the lived paradox of the human–companion animal bond. Doctoral Thesis. School of Health, Psychology and Social Care, Manchester Metropolitan University, Manchester, UK, pp. 380, 395–400, 415, 428.

Dawson SE (2007b) Companion animal bereavement. The Society of Practising Veterinary Surgeons' Review, pp. 31–32.

Dawson SE, Fowler J, Ormerod E, Sheridan E (2007) New perspectives on bonding. *Veterinary Review* 132:30–33.

Egan G (1986) *The Skilled Helper*. Brooks/Cole, Monterey, CA.

Kohut H (1971) *The Analysis of Self*. International Universities Press, New York.

Lagoni L, Butler C, Hetts S (1994) *The Human–Animal Bond and Grief*. Saunders, Philadelphia, PA, p. 32.

Lagoni L, Morehead D, Brannan J (2001) *Guidelines for Bond-Centred Practice*. Colorado State University, CO.

Lambert A (2006) *Missing My Pet*. BGTF, Horbling, Lincs, UK.

Meyers B (2000) Anticipatory mourning and the human–animal bond. In: Rando TA (ed.), *Clinical Dimension of Anticipatory Mourning: Theory and Practice in Working with the Dying, Their Loved Ones and Their Caregivers*. Research Press, Champaign, IL, p. 549.

Parkes CM (2006) *Love and Loss: The Roots of Grief and Its Complications*. Routledge, London, p. 1.

Rando TA (ed.) (1986) *Loss and Anticipatory Grief*. Lexington Books, Lexington, ID.

Stewart M (1999) *Companion Animal Death*. Butterworth-Heinemann, Oxford, pp. 38–39.

Stratton P, Hayes N (1999) *A Student's Dictionary of Psychology*. Arnold, London, pp. 74, 90.

Thompson TL (1986) *Communication for Health Professionals*. Harper and Row, New York.

Wilson EO (1993) Biophilia and the conservation ethic. In: Kellert SR, Wilson EO (eds), *The Biophilia Hypothesis*. Island Press/Shearwater Books, Washington, DC, p. 31.

Dealing with difficult situations

Carol Gray and Jenny Moffett

Introduction

In this chapter, we look at difficult situations that occur in veterinary practice, and how good communication can make a difference. We cover financial aspects of practice, dealing with 'informed' clients, dealing with anger, dealing with mistakes and communication in end-of-life situations.

THE USE OF VETERINARY COMMUNICATION SKILLS AT THE END-OF-LIFE

It has been said that the one thing that we can be sure of in life is death. And for those who work in general veterinary practice – and are involved in everything from the killing of farm animals for meat, through to the euthanasia of a much-loved pet – the death of their animal patients is a regular occurrence.

Some deaths are, however, more stressful to the client and vet than others – notably the death of animals to which clients have formed an emotional bond. In this section we concentrate on the issues surrounding the loss of a companion animal such as a dog or cat. However, most, if not all, of the communication techniques described below will be equally applicable to larger companion animals such as horses and ponies, or other species to which clients have become attached.

Whether the death of a companion animal comes after the result of a long and happy life or following an accident or a distressing illness, there are several communication techniques that can help both the client and the veterinary team cope with this stressful time. In this section we look at the difficulties associated with 'end-of-life' communication and evidence from the medical and veterinary literature as to best practice in this area.

Difficulties associated with end-of-life communication

Talking about death and other end-of-life topics can be difficult, and significant barriers to end-of-life communication have been identified in both the medical and veterinary literature (Curtis & Patrick 1997; Larson & Tobin 2000; Shaw & Lagoni 2007; Tinga et al. 2001). The death of a companion animal, whether by natural causes or as a result of euthanasia, can involve many emotionally charged issues, including unfavourable prognoses, treatment failures, time constraints, unease with death or dying, financial dilemmas and difficult decision making (Larson & Tobin 2000; Shaw & Lagoni 2007). Here, we investigate the issues which may affect the client and the vet at such times.

Client factors

There is some debate as to whether people experience the same type and duration of grief when a pet dies, as when a human companion dies. A study by Adams et al. (1999), for example, found that the grieving experience for most owners was 'short and practical as daily demands took over'. Participants in this study said that although they felt 'extremely sad' at the loss of their pet, their experience was 'not marked by the depth of depression that is often experienced when a human companion dies' (Adams et al. 1999).

However, that is not to say that clients do not grieve and suffer when a pet dies – the death of animal can have adverse psychological, emotional and even physical effects on owners (Adams et al. 1999, 2000; Hart et al. 1990). One study (Adams et al. 2000) found that approximately 30% of clients experienced 'severe grief' at the death of their companion animal.

Further to this, there is the suggestion that owners' expressions of grief at the loss of a pet may be 'truncated' because of the perception that it is not permissible to grieve for an animal (Adams et al. 1999). Owners have said that they struggled with the 'contradiction between how they felt after their pet had died and the perceived absence of support for their feelings from others, or society in general' (Adams et al. 1999).

It is also true to say that different people react to a companion animal's death in different ways. There are countless factors that contribute to this variability, including the client's personal beliefs, their stage of life, how demanding their job is and their previous exposure to a pet or human death (Adams et al. 1999, 2000). In some cases an owner may be so attached to their pet that they may be reluctant to permit euthanasia, even where it is required, in the best interest of the animal (Wensley 2008).

Beyond sadness, the loss of a loved one can also trigger other emotions such as anger and guilt (Hart et al. 1990; Shaw & Lagoni 2007; Weissman 2004). In one investigation into owners' attitudes to the euthanasia of their pet, 45% of the participants reported feeling guilty about making the decision to euthanize, whilst 16% said that they felt like a 'murderer' (Adams et al. 2000). Add to this emotional backdrop, we often ask clients to make the difficult decisions under time-limited circumstances, and we can see why end-of-life communication can be so traumatic for clients. Susan Elizabeth Dawson covers this area in much greater detail in Chapter 4.

Veterinary factors

It is not just clients that find end-of life discussions difficult. Evidence from the medical and veterinary literature reveals that health care professionals also find this a challenging area (Amiel et al. 2006; Hart & Hart 1987; Hart et al. 1990; Silverman et al. 2005; Tinga et al. 2001). When it comes to breaking bad news to clients, for example, it is clear that many professionals feel underconfident and inadequately trained (Amiel et al. 2006; Girgis & Sanson-Fisher 1998; Schmid Mast et al. 2005; Silverman et al. 2005; Tinga et al. 2001).

This is a worrying thought as, at least in the medical literature, there is an abundance of evidence to suggest that how bad news is communicated can have real and adverse effects on the patient and his or her family (Girgis & Sanson-Fisher 1998; Lowden 1998; Schmid Mast et al. 2005). Although there is a relative lack of veterinary-specific research in this area, it is likely that breaking bad news in a poor, or inappropriate, manner will have a negative effect on the owner of an animal to whom the bad news pertains.

Other examples of end-of-life communication, such as the euthanasia appointment, have been documented as having either positive or negative effects on clients (Adams et al. 1999). As Adams et al. (2000) say:

> It is unclear whether a supportive veterinarian can modify the duration or magnitude of grief reactions, or make clients feel better about a pet's death. However, it is likely that supportive veterinarians actually validate and normalize their client's reactions which, in turn, gives clients permission to grieve. Negative experiences at a veterinary practice certainly impact owners' responses.

It has also been reported that, in equine practice, more than 65% of client loss may be traced to insensitive handling of the euthanasia process (Brackenridge & Shoemaker 1996). All these factors generate extra pressure on a veterinarian who may be facing other issues at the end of an animal's life, such as their own attachment to the animal, their own experiences with loss (Lagoni et al. 1994) and the possibility that the loss of the patient could somehow equate to a personal failure (Weissman 2004).

A SEVEN-STEP APPROACH TO COMMUNICATION AT THE END-OF-LIFE

End-of-life communication covers a wide range of veterinary situations and experiences. Because of this, it is important to recognize that a 'one size fits all' approach to cases and clients does not work. However, during times of end-of-life communication, such as breaking bad news, relationship-centred models of communication have been highlighted as the most successful course of action (Schmid Mast et al. 2005). In this section, we look at how to impart bad news using a relationship-centred model of communication in conjunction with the seven-step communication tool of von Gunten et al. (2000), which imposes structure and a logical progression on the proceedings. This approach involves the following steps:

1. Prepare for the discussion.
2. Establish what the client (and family) knows.
3. Determine how information is to be handled.

4. Deliver the information.
5. Respond to emotions.
6. Establish goals for care and treatment priorities.
7. Establish a plan.

Preparation for the discussion

When you know you have bad news to impart to a client, it is important to prepare how you will impart that information. Identify who needs to be involved in the discussion (ask yourself, 'Who makes the decisions in this family?' and 'Does the client need moral support?') and then arrange a face-to-face consultation (Girgis & Sanson-Fisher 1998; Weissman 2004). When it comes to breaking bad news or serious discussions, avoid doing this over the telephone where at all possible (von Gunten et al. 2000).

Make sure you have established the facts of the case by looking at notes and discussing the case with other members of the veterinary team who have been involved. Then, choose an appropriate environment to hold the consultation – a quiet and private room is best (von Gunten et al. 2000; Ptacek & Ptacek 2001). Prepare the room by adding chairs and removing any barriers between where you and the client(s) will sit. It is also useful to have facial tissues available in anticipation of tears.

Schedule the appointment so that you have enough time to complete the consultation and make sure that you have no interruptions (Billson & Tyrrell 2003; Girgis & Sanson-Fisher 1998).

Establish what the client knows

When meeting a client to discuss bad news, it is important to find out what has been happening since you last met (Silverman et al. 2005). Summarize where things have got to and what has happened since you last saw the animal (Silverman et al. 2005). Use open questions such as, 'How has she been since I saw you last?' Open questions can also be used to establish what the client's understanding of the animal's situation is to-date (von Gunten et al. 2000).

Determine how the information is to be handled

It is important to determine at an early stage how much, or how little, a client wants to know about their animal's situation. Medical patients can be divided into 'seekers' (around 80%) and 'avoiders' of information (Silverman et al. 2005). Seekers cope better when given more information by their doctor, whilst avoiders cope better with less. It is thought that some of the factors involved in this difference of attitude include ethnic background, level of education, gender and age (Benbasset et al. 1998; Girgis & Sanson-Fisher 1998).

The literature suggests, however, that the majority of patients and owners want to know about all treatment options prior to making a decision (Benbasset et al. 1998; Girgis & Sanson-Fisher 1998; Slater et al. 1996). Each client should be treated on a case-for-case basis, and one of the clearest ways to determine how much information to deliver is to ask the client directly (Girgis & Sanson-Fisher 1998; Silverman et al. 2005).

Deliver the information

When breaking bad news, it is good practice to give the client some warning that you have difficult information to impart – a 'warning shot' (Ptacek & Ptacek 2001; Silverman et al. 2005). This can be a non-verbal cue, for example, sitting the client down or using a private room or a verbal cue along the lines of: 'I'm afraid the news isn't as good as we had hoped'.

Deliver the information in a sensitive but straightforward manner, avoiding jargon or euphemisms (Girgis & Sanson-Fisher 1998; Larson & Tobin 2000). Do not overwhelm the client (Billson & Tyrrell 2003; Silverman et al. 2005) – break the information down into small chunks and allow them time to absorb the information. It may be necessary to repeat important points. Be aware of your body language: an open posture, with uncrossed legs and arms, is most suitable, as is achieving good eye contact with the client and sitting/standing at the same level.

The veterinarian should neither overstate nor understate the implications of the news (von Gunten et al. 2000). Experts recommend 'hoping for the best but preparing for the worst' (Schmid Mast et al. 2005; Tulsky 2005; Weissman 2004) or, as Silverman et al. (2005) call it: 'hope tempered with realism'.

Fundamentally, though, the information should be truthful. As Weissman (2004) says, truthful information 'is often the single most important piece of information that patients need to make informed choices'. Specific prognostic information and the range of possible outcomes should also be discussed at this stage (von Gunten et al. 2000).

Respond to emotions

Bad news can trigger a wide range of emotional reactions for clients (von Gunten et al. 2000). One major example is 'anticipatory grief', a grief reaction that occurs in anticipation of an impending loss (Casarett et al. 2001). The veterinarian needs to be able to read and respond to such reactions empathetically. The veterinarian should aim to convey respect, acceptance and support to the client and can achieve this by using communication techniques such as active listening, questioning and paraphrasing (Larson & Tobin 2000). Non-verbal cues can also be used to convey warmth and reassurance, such as good eye contact, facing the patient, nodding encouragingly, giving full attention and not interrupting or writing notes while the client is talking (Girgis & Sanson-Fisher 1998; Silverman et al. 2005). It is also important to use pauses and silence – the client needs time and space to respond (Billson & Tyrrell 2003; Girgis & Sanson-Fisher 1998; Silverman et al. 2005).

Tulsky (2005) recommends attending to the client by following these five steps:

1. Acknowledge the emotion: 'This must be difficult news to take in'
2. Identify loss: 'I bet it's hard to imagine life without Snowy'
3. Legitimize the feelings: 'It's quite common for someone in this situation to have a hard time in making decisions'
4. Offer support: 'Whatever lies ahead, I will be here to help you'
5. Explore: 'You mentioned feeling angry. Can you tell me more about this?'

Again, Chapter 4 deals with client emotions in greater detail.

Establish goals for care and treatment priorities

Key to this relationship-centred model is that clients must sense that their ideas, feelings, expectations and fears are understood (Epstein et al. 1993) and that they are being actively involved in the decision-making process.

A review of the available medical literature (Larson & Tobin 2000) shows that human patients and their families, when facing a life-threatening illness, value the following: clear communication about the patient's condition, effective symptomatic management, preservation of autonomy and a sense of control, and the avoidance of a prolonged death. It is likely that some of these can be extrapolated to a veterinary situation. Open-ended questions such as, 'What would you like to see happening?', 'What's important to you now?' or 'What are you hoping for?', should help you to elicit a client's goals for his or her animal.

If, say, the discussion is likely to involve euthanasia as an option, you may want to use this occasion to explore the client's ideas of quality of life for their pet. According to Wojciechowska and Hewson (2005), veterinarians can accurately assess a dog's physical health but they cannot easily ascertain the dog's mental well-being – it is down to the client to provide information about the dog's experience and perspective as they are most familiar with his or her personality, behaviour and daily routine.

Note, however, that some people may be so overwhelmed with the initial bad news that they will not be able to discuss goals and this must be done at a later session (von Gunten et al. 2000).

Establish a plan

Once you and the client have discussed the situation, the next step is to establish a plan for future events. If possible, do not rush the client into any decisions – follow-up meetings or telephone calls can be scheduled if required. In addition, clients can be supplied with more information (reading material, videos, etc.) on their animal's condition or, say, on euthanasia (Girgis & Sanson-Fisher 1998).

Remember that, at this stage, reassurance is also important. Clients will want to know that, despite the bad news, they are not being 'abandoned' (Larson & Tobin 2000; Weissman 2004). It may help to gently remind them that you also want the best care for the patient and to reinforce that you are working with the client to achieve this (von Gunten et al. 2000).

Summarize what you have discussed and check that the client is OK with the arrangements. After the consultation, you should document the information you have given to the client, as well as discuss the proceedings with other relevant members of staff (Billson & Tyrrell 2003; Girgis & Sanson-Fisher 1998; Silverman et al. 2005).

EUTHANASIA – BEFORE, DURING AND AFTER

The euthanasia appointment is the commonest point where veterinary professionals interact with clients at the end of an animal's life. It can be an unpleasant, and unfortunately frequent, task. However, it is also a veterinary duty that, if handled competently and sensitively, can be one of the best ways of cementing a veterinary–client relationship. As the old adage goes, 'clients don't care how much you know until they know how much you care'.

Euthanasia – before

A pre-euthanasia appointment is highly recommended. At this appointment, you will be able to discuss the procedure and the choices that the client will have.

First, by explaining the procedure and what to expect, the client can make a decision as to whether they want to be present at the euthanasia or not. It has been reported that vets may be against offering client-present euthanasia because of such factors as time limitations, having to deal with clients' emotions and their own emotions, or the fear that something may go wrong with the procedure (Lagoni et al. 1994; Tinga et al. 2001). However, it is important that clients have been given the choice to be present or not (Adams et al. 1999; Hart et al. 1990; Lagoni et al. 1994; Martin et al. 2004) – in one study, 70% of owners said that they wanted the option to be present (Adams et al. 2000). Witnessing a peaceful euthanasia can help clients come to terms with the death, but it is important that it is their decision – be careful not to talk a client into being present if they do not want to (Lagoni et al. 1994).

Second, you can ascertain if the client wants to have the euthanasia carried out at home. A home euthanasia is often the least stressful option for an animal or owner, especially where the animal is very old, sick or debilitated.

Third, offer the choices for cremation and burial. Clients are often unaware of what happens to an animal's body after death and what each choice of disposal entails (Hart et al. 1990). It is necessary to be honest about what happens to an animal's body in each instance. In one anecdotal report, Lagoni et al. (1994) talk of an elderly woman who decided to let her veterinarian dispose of her dog's body. The woman was told that the dog was being buried in a 'mass grave' and the dog's body went to a local landfill site. However, the vet was left in a tricky situation a month later when the woman returned to enquire about the grave's location so that she could visit her pet's final resting place.

Fourth, plan the logistics of the euthanasia – make an appointment and enquire whether the client would like to sign the consent form and pay the bill in advance (Lagoni et al. 1994). On leaving, the client can be offered pet loss support reading material or videos/DVDs.

Euthanasia – during

A euthanasia appointment should, where possible, be scheduled for a quiet time of day, such as at lunchtime or after hours (Hart et al. 1990). When clients arrive for such an appointment, they should be ushered straight into the consulting room and not left in the waiting room (Hart et al. 1990). At this stage, you can discuss the procedure with the client again, offering options and confirming choices (Hart et al. 1990). Ask clients if they want a little time alone with their pet before the procedure. Make sure you have someone to help you restrain the animal and raise the vein. Take any consulting room phones off the hook, turn off pagers or mobile phones and talk to the practice reception staff to make sure that you are not interrupted during the procedure.

Have all of your necessary equipment ready, including the needles and syringes, and clip and prep the animal for injection. Some authors recommend pre-placement of a catheter in either the cephalic or the saphenous vein (Hart et al. 1990) – remember, in this instance, to use heparin flush before introducing the euthanasia solution. In some older, sicker animals you will not be able to do so. You should warn the client of this and that it may be difficult to locate a vein. In other cases, sedation or tranquilization of an animal may be required. At this point, you can remind the client of the bodily reactions, which should have been brought up at the pre-euthanasia appointment. Reactions to discuss include bladder and bowel evacuation, twitching muscles, failure of eyes to close and the fact that the pet may call out or gasp deeply on death.

After injecting the solution, allow the animal to sink to the table gently and then use your stethoscope to check there is no heartbeat. Simply state that the animal is dead. At this point, touch, such as resting your hand gently on the client's arm, can be an effective way of expressing compassion (Hart et al. 1990). Be aware, however, of cultural differences or individual attitudes.

During the euthanasia consultation, what you do and say, and how you do and say it, are important indicators to the client as to the significance of the situation (Adams et al. 1999). Ideally, a client should feel comfortable enough to express emotion in front of the veterinary team. Although clients do not expect their vet to provide counselling skills (Adams et al. 1999), they do at least deserve to receive a level of compassion and understanding.

Specifically, Lagoni et al. (1994) recommend the following:

- Acknowledging that the pet has died: do not be afraid to talk about it.
- Normalizing the situation for the client: lend credibility to their feelings, behaviours, experiences and thoughts – allow the owner to cry without feeling embarrassed (Adams et al. 1999).
- Giving permission: encourage clients to voice their needs and wishes without fear of judgement

Avoid clichés such as 'I know how you feel', 'He had a long life', or switching to your own thoughts, 'When my dog died . . .'. Instead, use open-ended questions and exploring statements to encourage the client to open up about their own feelings and perceptions; for example, 'Tell me a bit about Sooty . . .'. Most veterinary communication experts advise against recommending obtaining another pet during the euthanasia consultation (Hart et al. 1990; Lagoni et al. 1994).

Remember also that although some clients can appear abrupt or uncaring by veterinary staff, it may be that this is simply a strategy to retain control over their emotions in front of the veterinarian (Adams et al. 1999). It may also mean that the client is going through a form of shock or 'delayed grief'.

At this stage, the idea of counselling or pet loss support helplines can be introduced, where required (AVMA 2005; Hart et al. 1990). Chapter 4 has more information on these facilities.

Euthanasia – after

Ask the client if they would like time alone with their animal and give it to them. Even if the client is not present at the euthanasia, it is good practice to let them see the deceased animal (Hart et al. 1990). Present the body compassionately: clean up any blood, remove the catheter and place a bandage and cover with a blanket (von Gunten et al. 2000). Also, if they would

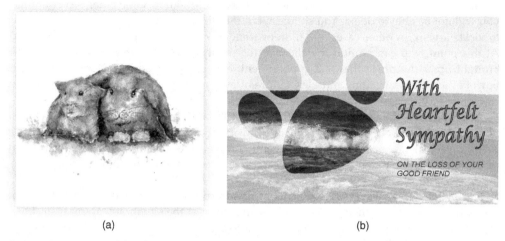

(a)   (b)

Figure 5.1 (a) Example of veterinary condolence card. Reproduced with the permission of Sarah Brown, Sarah Brown Cards. (b) Example of veterinary condolence card. Reproduced with kind permission from Pet-Urns.com.

like to clip a little fur or take the animal's collar, etc., then make sure they feel comfortable doing so.

If the owner is taking the animal home with them, do not handle the body roughly or awkwardly and make sure that you use appropriate coverings; anecdotally, clients do not want to receive their animal's body in a cardboard box or plastic bag (Lagoni et al. 1994). Also, if an animal goes for cremation, it is better to return ashes in a private room rather than across the desk in reception (Adams et al. 1999).

When clients are ready to leave, they should, where possible, be escorted out of a back or side door. Amend the animal's records and discuss the event with other staff so that the whole veterinary team is aware of the animal's deceased status. Follow-up letters and condolence cards (Figure 5.1) are often welcome additions to clients, but use your discretion and assess each client on a case-by-case basis – in one study, a few condolence card recipients were offended by this practice (Adams et al. 1999).

Euthanasia can be a sad and stressful time for the veterinarian. There has even been the suggestion that performing a large number of euthanasias can alter the veterinary professionals' attitude to mortality. Persaud (2007), for example, says that it is possible that vets can start to see death as 'a ready and available solution to problems'. In a study of how veterinarians handle euthanasias, the top stressors for vets were accidental deaths in their hospital, needless euthanasia of healthy animals or those that could have been saved with veterinary care and losses by long-term clients (Hart et al. 1990). Veterinary staff should also be wary of particularly demanding cases or several euthanasias carried out in a short space of time (Hart et al. 1990).

It is essential that veterinary professionals are aware of the ideas and emotions that euthanasia evoke within them. After a stressful euthanasia, it is necessary that vets are allowed to take time out and to acknowledge their reactions. They should not be afraid to grieve or to show emotion. A debriefing system or staff emotional support network is a good way to bringing challenging emotional situations out into the open. Further details on stress and coping mechanisms are provided in Chapter 8.

Summary

Death and dying are two of the most difficult topics for people – clients and veterinary professionals alike – to discuss. In the veterinary consultation this leads to a number of extra barriers to the communication process. However, there are several learned communication techniques and practices which can help. An example is the seven-step approach to communication at end of life. This includes preparing for the discussion, establishing what the client (and family) knows, determining how information is to be handled, delivering the information, responding to emotions, establishing goals for care and treatment priorities and establishing a plan. Euthanasia consultations are a major example of where to put these communication skills into operation.

WELFARE CONCERNS

An area of difficult communication for any veterinary professional is when there is concern over animal welfare. This could include neglect (e.g. failure to treat a condition until it becomes untreatable), prolonging treatment when euthanasia would be in the animal's best interests and non-accidental injury (NAI).

If an animal is showing signs of neglect, the veterinary surgeon should try to find out from the client what has been happening. For example, a client brings in an extremely thin dog. The veterinary professional must hide any shock or temptation to blame the client for the animal's condition, and instead try to get the client to discuss the problem:

> He's not looking very happy, and I'm worried about his weight – can you take me through what has been happening with him?

A team approach to caring for a suspected case of neglect may turn things around with dietary advice, regular weighing and routine investigations to see if there is an explanation for the weight loss; this may be enough to deal with it.

Other cases where 'neglect' is a factor include rabbits with blowfly strike (maggots), grossly obese dogs or cats and severe cases of flea-allergic skin irritation. It is sometimes difficult to avoid apportioning blame, but trying to look forward rather than backward will often work.

> It's good that you have brought him along to the practice now, and we will work together to try to make things better as quickly as possible.

If the condition has progressed so far that euthanasia is the only treatment option from a welfare perspective, the veterinary surgeon must act as advocate for the animal:

> We really can't do any more for him; I'm so sorry – we need to do what's best for him and let him go now.

If the client refuses to agree to euthanasia, one option for the veterinary surgeon involved is to get a second opinion from a colleague at the practice. If this does not persuade the client of the correct course of action, what can the veterinary surgeon do? If it is not possible to supply pain relief to keep the animal comfortable while the client makes a decision, then the veterinary surgeon must sometimes make the difficult decision to get an animal welfare authority involved (Morgan & McDonald 2007). This is, of course, a last resort, as the veterinary surgeon–client relationship may not recover from such an action. The veterinary surgeon would have to be sure that there was no other option.

It is suspected that NAI is under-reported in veterinary practice. In a study undertaken by Munro and Thrusfield (2001), 48.3% of respondents had suspected or seen cases of NAI. Suspicions are aroused if an animal's injuries do not correspond with the owner's description of how they occurred, or if there are discrepancies in the history between members of the family. The fact that an animal has been abused should be enough motivation for the veterinary surgeon to want to do something to prevent it happening again, but there is an even bigger motivation with the well-documented links with child abuse and domestic violence.

Mandatory reporting of suspected NAI has been advocated for the veterinary profession in the United Kingdom, but the Royal College of Veterinary Surgeons (RCVS) view is that its current guidelines are sufficient (Anon 2007). However, it is a legal requirement in some states of the USA (Babcock & Neihsl 2006). This is one of the occasions when client confidentiality can be breached.

So, how would 'gathering information' work if a veterinary surgeon suspected a case of NAI? One approach would be to ask: 'I'm still not clear how the injuries were caused – could you go back over what happened again?'

In this case, the vet would not summarize the history to check with the client, but would be looking for inconsistencies in the repeated narrative. Obviously, it would be necessary to get enough information to confirm suspicions. Would it also be necessary to avoid arousing suspicion in the client? Probably not, as if this does turn out to be a case of NAI, the veterinarian–client relationship would be irretrievably damaged anyway. If it does not turn out to be the case, then the client would probably not even notice the way the questioning was carried out.

INFORMED CLIENTS

A particular area of difficulty for communication seems to be when dealing with informed clients (Figure 5.2). We are mainly talking about two different types of client here – those with knowledge gained through experience (farmers, horse owners, clients with the same disease as their pet or who have someone close to them with the same disease, dog and cat

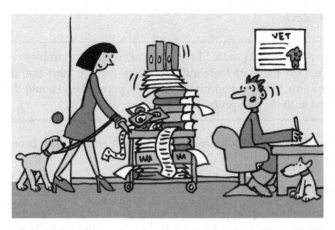

Figure 5.2   The informed client.

breeders) and those with knowledge gained through their own research (increasingly, this means knowledge gained by searching the internet).

Why do such clients pose problems for veterinary surgeons? This may hark back to the 'old days' of paternalistic veterinary practice. The veterinary surgeon knew best and there was no discussion with the client, merely giving them instructions for what would happen next. There may have been a feeling that keeping clients in ignorance kept them bound to the veterinary surgeon in a dependent relationship (Waldsmith 2003). These veterinary surgeons must have been shocked when clients started answering back, or asking questions, or disagreeing with a plan of action. In fact, 'informed' clients should be a common aim for every consultation, and if they have done their own research or bring their own experience to the table, surely that should make the veterinary professional's job easier? Rather than having to explain findings or plans in great detail, he/she merely has to check that the client's information is correct, and temper any explanations accordingly.

For example, a new client brings in an elderly cat, and hands the veterinary surgeon a stack of printed pages with information about renal disease in cats: 'I know what's wrong with Tinkerbell – it's her kidneys'.

An initial temptation to take the pile of paper and put it straight in the bin must be resisted. Instead, the veterinary surgeon needs to become part of the team involved in the cat's care.

> Well, Mrs Client – I am very encouraged by your enthusiasm for researching Tinkerbell's condition, and you may well be right. Let's have a chat about what has been happening with her, and then we'll have a look at her and see if everything points towards kidney problems, and we'll take it from there.

After taking a thorough history and examining the cat, the vet is more convinced that the cat is hyperthyroid. The client still needs to feel involved, however, and this can be achieved by directing her research:

> So, as we've discussed, it looks more likely that Tinkerbell has a problem with her thyroid gland. I've written the name of the condition down for you, and also the addresses of some reliable websites. While we admit her for tests, perhaps you could do some research on caring for a cat with thyroid problems.

This should result in a client who feels part of the team, and has been credited for her research rather than feeling belittled.

Informed client groups

There has been a move in medical practice to create so-called expert patients, who are more involved in the management and treatment of their own disease by being given access to educational materials to help them to understand their condition. It would seem sensible that such a scheme would lend itself to veterinary practice, with 'support groups' being set up in each practice for common conditions, where clients, led by a member of the practice team, would help each other to cope with the problems of caring for an animal with that condition. However, the 'expert patient' scheme has had mixed reactions, and the initial fear that such patients would take up more physician time (Shaw & Baker 2004) has been proved correct in several studies looking at lay-led programmes (Griffiths et al. 2007). It seems that a support scheme led by a professional, such as would occur with the suggested mode of delivery in veterinary practice, is actually more effective (Griffiths et al. 2007).

COMMUNICATING COST

Financial discussions are often problematic for veterinary surgeons. It is not difficult to understand why this should be the case. In a Canadian study on how pet owners and practitioners view monetary issues (Coe et al. 2007) one participant remarked:

> [P]et owners view those working in the veterinary profession as being there out of a genuine love for and interest in animals, rather than for strict monetary gain.

This can lead to a feeling of being undervalued, certainly in small animal practice. This feeling can be exacerbated by the tendency of practice principals to underprice services such as neutering and vaccination in order to compete with neighbouring practices.

However, the same has happened in large animal practice, where the emphasis has traditionally been on supply of drugs and vaccines, so the veterinary surgeons:

> ... practically gave away their time and expertise just to sell these other things. (Whitford 2004).

This does not mean that the veterinary profession is alone in being reticent about discussing costs. A study to determine how well the medical profession copes with this has been conducted in the USA, where physicians discussed costs and/or insurance with only 12% of patients prescribed new medication (Tarn et al. 2006). They were also more likely to discuss costs with patients earning less than $20 000 annually.

So, how do we discuss costs with clients? One suggestion is that they should be discussed with specific reference to the animal's health and prognosis (Coe et al. 2007). We should not feel embarrassed about proposing expensive treatment options, provided they are in the best interests of the animal, so that what we are actively selling is good welfare (Main 2006). However, in some cases this may mean advocating the treatment that is least profitable for the practice (euthanasia). If the animal's welfare is always used as the basis for decision making, it is difficult to see how the client would get the impression that the practice was interested only in profit. For example, if the veterinary surgeon decides that the proposed best treatment option is beyond the capability of the primary care practice, then referral should be offered, with the reasons why the vet feels that this is the best option. This is more likely to bring the client back to the primary care practice after specialist treatment than to result in a request for permanent transfer. Contrast this with the situation where the client requests referral due to dissatisfaction with the primary care practice, which is less likely to result in the client returning (Osborne 2002).

This approach could impact on veterinary surgeons working for practices where ATV (average transaction per vet) is the sole criterion for success. The pressure to 'sell' products and services that may not be in the animal's best interests may cause ethical problems for members of the practice team. As Osborne (2001) observed, there is:

> ... an ethical difference between the motive behind generating value-based free enterprise fees-for-service needed to maintain the fiscal vitality of properly staffed and equipped veterinary hospitals, and the motive behind peddling unnecessary services and products to increase fees to a maximum determined by what the traffic will bear.

Each individual must make a decision about whether to continue working for such practices, if this type of business approach causes discomfort.

Raising the subject of cost should be an integral part of explaining and planning with the client. Clients should never have to bring up the subject of costs; they should be included in the cost–benefit analysis used by the veterinary surgeon to aid in decision making. Signposting should indicate to the client that costs will be discussed. For example:

There are three options for treating this condition, with a range of costs associated with them. I will take you through each one in turn, and you can ask if you need more information on anything as we go through them.

We may have an answer to why so many veterinary surgeons find it difficult to charge properly for their services. As a nation renowned for caring for animals, we feel that there should be a 'collective responsibility' for animal care, and that veterinary surgeons choose their career because of an overwhelming interest in animal welfare rather than financial reward. This latter fact would appear to be true, as annual income for veterinary surgeons compares unfavourably with figures for other health professions; for example for 2007, an average annual salary of £78 882 for medical practitioners compared with an average of £36 335 for veterinary surgeons (GMB 2007).

Of course, the other compelling argument is that animals are their owners' property, luxuries rather than necessities, and owners must take on the responsibility of paying for treatment when they decide to own animals. There has long been a movement to bring back dog licences in Great Britain (they are already restored in Northern Ireland) since their abolition in 1987, or to have some sort of qualification for owning animals. This may emphasize the financial responsibility involved.

Does waiving fees, or undercharging for services provided, actually do the profession any good? It may be that *not* charging appropriate fees gives veterinary surgeons a higher standing as far as public opinion is concerned, but it also means that the ongoing, fixed costs of running a practice may not be met. Some veterinary surgeons make their clients aware of the running costs involved ('it costs £xxxx per day just to keep the surgery open'), but should we really have to justify the fees charged in such detail? Does this not devalue the profession? Clients should be willing to pay a fair price for the service provided because they are receiving a professional service (Klingborg & Klingborg 2007).

Clients with private medical insurance may appreciate the cost of surgical procedures, as they are used to the itemized billing for private medical care. For example, with the average cost of a hysterectomy in private hospitals in the UK being £4–5000, a bill of £350 for a similar procedure in a large-breed dog will not seem unreasonable. However, with most clients using the NHS for their own treatment, they will not be aware of the sort of costs involved in, for example, general anaesthesia or surgical time. It is extremely important to provide an itemized bill for all surgical or in-patient procedures so that the client is aware of how the bill is calculated (RCVS 2008). Obviously, the client should be given an estimated cost of any procedure beforehand, as part of the informed consent process (see Chapter 3).

One solution that has been proposed is to use 'estimate sheets' with the costs involved for all of the most common conditions presented in practice. These sheets then become an integral part of every decision-making discussion (Milani 2003).

What is the difference between a quote and an estimate? A quote is a fixed price for an agreed service, while an estimate is an approximate price based on what the 'expert' believes will have to be done to remedy the problem. As the study by Coe et al. (2007) discovered, '. . . vets view them as estimates, and clients view them as quotes . . .'.

Estimates are approximations, but sometimes veterinary surgeons use them as an excuse to keep adding to a bill without informing a client of what is happening. Is this ethical? No. According to the RCVS, clients should be kept informed of running totals, and their consent given before adding to the bill (RCVS 2008).

For example, a dog is hospitalized for investigation and treatment of a suspected heart condition. The estimate of £250 for initial work-up is reached on day 2, and there are still tests that the vet would like to perform. The client is contacted by telephone:

Mrs Anderson – we are phoning you to bring you up-to-date with Bruno's progress. He's had a comfortable night, and is eating a little better. He had about half of his normal meal this morning. His heart condition is stable, but we are still worried about the fluid build-up in his chest. We'd like to do some more investigations to see if we can safely drain this fluid, to make him more comfortable, but I'm afraid that will add another £150 to the bill. Would you be willing for us to go ahead? If not, we can keep him on the water pills to try to get rid of the fluid, and we would hope that these drugs would remove it, but it may take a few days. Your current treatment bill is £239.

What about pet insurance? The effect of prepaid health plans has been studied in the medical profession in the USA. Bradley and Gehlbach (1988) found that such plans actually improved clinical decision making, but also increased the number of patient visits.

It is suggested that the people who really need pet insurance are the least likely to have it (Roen 2001). One view is that veterinary surgeons should inform clients at first visits (e.g. with a new puppy or kitten) of the true cost of veterinary treatment (Montgomery 2001). It is suggested that this could be achieved by members of the practice team giving clients an example of one common disease and one accidental injury, with detailed costs breakdown for each, and a recommendation that they take out insurance. However, it is impossible to predict how much an owner is prepared to spend on an animal, and lack of insurance should never limit the treatment options presented, no matter how expensive they may be.

Often, the most difficult conversations take place when the owner cannot afford to have the animal treated, and opts for euthanasia. This is common in equine practice, happens frequently with small pets, and is increasingly a dilemma with cancer treatment of companion animals. In this situation, the euthanasia option should be presented as a valid 'treatment' option, not as a last resort. Saying to the client that 'these are the options for treatment, and the only other thing we can do is put him to sleep' will increase feelings of guilt if the client has to choose euthanasia as the only affordable option. Sometimes, the best welfare option will involve euthanasia of the animal, and as the advocate for animal welfare, the veterinary surgeon should make sure that this option is among the first given.

DEALING WITH ANGER

A common 'heart-sink' type of client for veterinary surgeons is the angry client (Figure 5.3). Indeed, many of our undergraduate veterinary students find dealing with angry clients the most difficult challenge for them during communication skills training sessions.

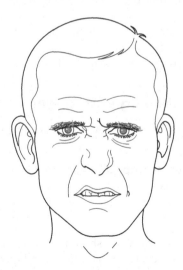

Figure 5.3 The angry client.

Angry clients may not be able to communicate their concerns effectively, are more likely to be non-compliant and may be more likely to sue over minor mishaps (McCord et al. 2002).

In medicine, one study found that physicians rated greater than 15% of patients as 'difficult', with the result that they felt uneasy and hoped that such patients would not return for follow-up visits (Jackson & Kroenke 1999). Often, the problem with these patients is unmet expectations, with most of these related to physician communication (33% of patients had unmet expectations concerning diagnosis, and 51% had unmet expectations concerning prognosis) rather than physician action, such as prescription of a medication, appointment for a diagnostic test or referral to a specialist (Jackson & Kroenke 2001). It would seem logical that a first step in dealing with them is to find out what their expectations were, how they were unmet, and how this made them feel. Lazoritz (2004) suggests asking the questions, giving the patient a 'magic minute' without interrupting, listening to the responses, and then asking, 'What would make you feel better?'

Using empathy

Empathy is an effective strategy when dealing with anger, although when faced with an angry client, it may be the most difficult tool to fetch from the toolbox.

An empathic response 'accurately identifies the factual content . . . as well as the nature and intensity of . . . feelings, concerns or quandaries' (Coulehan et al. 2001).

Platt and Keller (1994) advise the following strategy:

1. Be aware – listen for strong feelings.
2. Reflect – identify the feeling internally: 'This client sounds angry'.
3. Name the feeling – you may get it wrong, but the client will correct you. Do not rush into further explanations or treatment – just be with the client: 'It sounds like you are very angry about this'.
4. Make sense of the feeling – ask for an explanation if it does not make sense: 'I can tell that you feel strongly about this, but I'm not sure if I understand exactly how you feel – can you tell me?'
5. Affirm the feeling – summarize what has made the client angry, then add, 'Yes, I can see how that would make you feel angry'.
6. Offer help – 'Let's see what we can do to make this better'.

A practical guide for dealing with anger

Wasan et al. (2005) suggest 'Five 'As' for dealing with hostile patients:

1. Acknowledge the problem
2. Allow the patient to vent uninterrupted in a private place
3. Agree on what the problem is
4. Affirm what can be done
5. Assure follow-up

So, if we have an angry client to deal with, should we aim for a similar protocol? There is nothing to suggest that there are fundamental differences between angry clients and angry patients, or any other type of angry individual. We need to deal with the emotion (anger) to enable the person to rationalize what has happened and to try to move forward to a possible solution.

Our first step should be to take the client into a private room – an office or a consulting room would be suitable. This acknowledges that they are upset about something. There should be two chairs available and the client should be offered a seat. If they do not wish to sit down, it is often an effective strategy for the veterinary professional to sit down and to continue to offer the client a seat. Removing one person to a lower level than the other is an effective non-verbal cue that may result in lowering the anger level.

Next, the client should be invited to explain why they are angry, and the veterinary professional should shut up and listen, using 'active' or empathic listening. Sometimes this can be enough to dissipate anger on its own, but it also introduces an aura of respect and concern, which may be enough to encourage the angry individual to reflect similar attitudes (Egan 1975).

The veterinary professional should periodically summarize, to check back on the details, and should also use empathic statements:

Let me see if I have got this right (a clarifying statement to introduce the summary)
I can imagine how you might have felt (empathic statement)
Is there anything else? (screening)

The next step is to ask the client what they think should happen next: 'How can we make this better for you?' The client's demands may be unrealistic, but at least there is now a starting point for resolution. Note-taking during the meeting also validates the client's concerns. Finally, give the client a point of contact in the practice to keep them updated on the progress of their complaint, and keep them informed, preferably in writing.

Apologizing is usually an effective technique for dealing with anger, but it needs to be done correctly.

What works best to dissipate anger?

In one of the few studies looking at effective techniques for dealing with anger, where patients were angry due to being kept waiting, ownership of the apology ('I apologize for your long wait') was rated significantly higher than apology without ownership ('I'm sorry that you have been kept waiting'). If this apology was accompanied by an explanation for the wait, it scored even higher. Following the apology and explanation, most patients wanted the follow-up questions to lead directly on to the medical interview rather than to an exploration of their feelings (McCord et al. 2002). So, it seems that apologizing with ownership of the problem, explaining why there was a problem, and then moving on to the reason for the visit were the most effective techniques for dealing with anger due to being kept waiting, a common cause of anger among users of health care services.

Other techniques to bear in mind when dealing with anger include non-confrontational body language and non-verbal behaviour. We have already mentioned trying to sit down and to get the client seated too. It is also useful to pay attention to tone of voice. It is easy to 'match' the client's tone of voice, but this is likely to inflame the situation. Try to keep your tone of voice lower and quieter than that of the client. Rate of speech is also important – a pause before answering any questions, and being deliberate over words used, acts to 'slow down' the ping-pong tendency of an angry exchange. We have already mentioned active and empathic listening. Maintain appropriate eye contact, which may be more difficult if you are taking notes, and encourage the client to speak by using facilitative responses, such as nodding and minimal expressions ('mmm', 'uh-huh').

Finally, remember that dealing with angry clients can be rewarding if you manage to resolve the situation to the satisfaction of both parties.

COMMUNICATION OF MISTAKES

'Everyone makes mistakes', 'You're only human!' It seems that part of the human condition is the ability to make mistakes and, whilst these may be shrugged off or smiled at under ordinary circumstances, they are no laughing matter in the context of our working lives. Yes, we all make mistakes, but that is of little comfort when faced with a severely ill, or dead, animal and the prospect of a lawsuit.

So, when we talk about errors or mistakes in a clinical situation, what do we mean? In the medical literature, Wu (2000) defines an error as:

> [A] commission or an omission with potentially negative consequences for the patient that would have been judged wrong by skilled and knowledgeable peers at the time it occurred, independent of whether there were any negative consequences.

In the USA, medical error results in 44 000–98 000 human deaths and 1 million injuries each year (Weingart et al. 2000). Studies have revealed that surgical mistakes are the most common form of error, but that complications from drug treatment, therapeutic mishaps and diagnostic errors can also occur (Weingart et al. 2000). What little work has been carried out in veterinary circles mirrors this variety of errors. In their survey of mistakes made by recent veterinary graduates, Mellanby and Herrtage (2004) found that:

> The most common mistakes involved the failure to perform an appropriate diagnostic test, surgical mistakes during non-neutering procedures and the administration of inappropriate drugs or medical treatment.

There are several factors that can help bring about medical or veterinary mistakes. These include errors of judgement, differences in species, poor communication, carelessness, as well as staff issues such as high workloads, inadequate supervision and limited knowledge or experience (Bonvicini et al. 2009; Rosner et al. 2000; Short 1994; Weingart et al. 2000). Mellanby and Herrtage (2004) discovered that 78% of recent graduates admitted to having made a mistake in their first years of practice. Of those that admitted to an error, and went on to describe the event in further detail, 74% cited their 'lack of experience' as a factor.

What do patients and veterinary clients want?

When an error in veterinary practice takes place, it is usually the animal that will bear any physical consequences. However, with 85% of small animal pet owners describing their pet as a 'family member', it is possible that a veterinary error may also have adverse emotional consequences for clients (Brown & Silverman 1999).

Medical research shows that patients who have experienced an error in their health care can feel a mixture of emotions, including sadness, anxiety, depression, anger and frustration (Gallagher et al. 2003). Furthermore, patients report that 'the way the error was disclosed to them directly affected their emotional experience of the error' (Gallagher et al. 2003).

After a mistake has occurred, patients want good communication with their doctor and information about what happened. Effective communication can make the difference being patients perceiving an error as 'an honest mistake' or as 'incompetence or malicious intent' (Duclos et al. 2005).

However, explanations alone do not necessarily result in patient satisfaction (Mazor et al. 2004). Patients also require an appreciation of the trauma they have suffered, assurances that lessons have been learned from their experiences and a genuine apology (Gallagher et al. 2003; Liang 2002; Vincent et al. 1994). According to Vincent et al. (1994), those who do not receive such information and assurances, or who feel they have been handled insensitively, are more likely to take legal action. This is supported by Forster et al. (2002), who say:

> When patients or their families are confronted by silence or evasion, they may see the threat of litigation as the only tool to rectify the imbalance of power and knowledge.

In contrast, those patients that had perceived good communication with their health care providers said that they felt less emotional trauma as a result of the mistake, were less likely to take legal action and were more likely to continue to see their doctor following the adverse event (Duclos et al. 2005; Vincent et al. 1994).

What do health care professionals provide?

We now have an idea of what patients want but, should an error occur, what do health care providers actually do? Much of the research has shown that health care providers do not always respond adequately to patients' needs following medical errors or complications (Duclos et al. 2005; Forster et al. 2002) and, in general, patients expect more detailed information than doctors believe they should give (Hingorani et al. 1999).

The medical literature strongly supports disclosure (Fein et al. 2007; Gallagher et al. 2003; Mazor et al. 2004; Rosner et al. 2000); the health care provider admits to an error whilst explaining its consequences, as well as why and how it happened. Full disclosure by health care providers is, however, uncommon (Gallagher et al. 2003). Research shows that, on average, only one in four medical errors is disclosed (Fein et al. 2007). In addition, clinicians are particularly reluctant to apologize when a mistake has occurred (Gallagher et al. 2003; Mazor et al. 2004).

There are several reasons why practitioners are reluctant to speak out following an error. These can include an attempt to protect patients from 'potentially detrimental anxiety', a fear of losing patients' trust, a fear of being sued and a fear of appearing incompetent or inadequate (Hingorani et al. 1999). In addition, practitioners can find disclosure a time-consuming, difficult and unpleasant task (Gallagher et al. 2003; Hingorani et al. 1999).

Although a fear of litigation is a legitimate fear for health care providers, it should be pointed out that much of the current research suggest that, paradoxically, a failure to provide patients with adequate information and an apology increases the risk of legal action (Forster et al. 2002; Gallagher et al. 2003; Hingorani et al. 1999). As Forster et al. (2002) say, 'When patients and their families are sad about the outcome but content with the doctoring, they are unlikely to ever set foot in a lawyer's office'.

The art of mistake communication

If we accept that making mistakes in veterinary practice is inevitable, we can propose that a measure of good communication can help install a 'safety net' in anticipation of an adverse event. We cannot prevent mistakes from happening but we can, as O'Connell and Bonvicini (2007) explain, '[Ensure] that clients have realistic expectations and understand the uncertainties in diagnosis and treatment'.

Should a veterinary practitioner make an error, there is a certain amount of professional guidance available. In the UK, for example, the RCVS (2008) advises that:

A sympathetic approach should be used in response to a complaint rather than immediate denial and defensiveness. An expression of sorrow that an animal has died or that someone is distressed by what has happened is appropriate and does not in itself amount to an admission of liability.

Similarly, the Veterinary Defence Society Ltd (2003) provides guidelines for coping with client complaints (Box 5.1), a frequent consequence of a clinical mistake.

Box 5.1 Guidelines for coping with client complaints

When a client complains to you in person or by phone, the most important thing is to make sure they feel you are really listening. If you can take the time and space to listen properly first time around, it may well save a lot of extra time and trouble later on.

Here are some useful tips to bear in mind:

- Stay calm.
- Take the client to a private, seated area or transfer their call to a quiet zone.
- Thank the client for bringing the matter to your attention.
- Ask them to tell you the full story from the beginning.
- Just listen and keep listening – do not interrupt or argue.
- Empathize – but it is generally better to avoid phrases such as 'I know how you feel' (you cannot).
- Pick up on key words e.g. 'You must have been very worried about X (pet's name)'.
- Take notes – and check the client agrees with what you have written.
- Summarize for the client what has been said to make sure you have not misunderstood or missed anything.

Say sorry and mean it

Once you have listened carefully, express regret that the client is dissatisfied. This is often all the client needs, but it must sound genuine. So:

- Be sincere – the person you are talking to will detect and resent an automatic response.
- Remember, an expression of regret will make the client feel heard and understood. It does not mean you are admitting liability – it simply means you are acknowledging the upset and are 'sorry that something has happened', not 'sorry it was caused by anyone's fault'.
- Try not to make apologies on behalf of someone else – or let someone else apologize for you. The client may feel fobbed off and could end up unhappier than before.
- Get the client on your side by saying things such as, 'How can *we* solve the problem?'

Explain quickly and clearly

A prompt and thorough explanation can work wonders too. Here are some key points that might help, most of which apply to written explanations too:

- Focus on the key issues the client is concerned about – and ask in what order they would like you to cover them.
- Use clear language and explain any veterinary jargon.
- Encourage the client to ask questions throughout.
- Check they have understood, for example 'I'm not sure I've put that clearly. Did that make sense?'
- Ask the client if your explanation has answered their concerns.
- Reassure them that the matter will be dealt with promptly and that you'll keep them informed of progress.
- To identify the specific issues of a complaint, it may be helpful to ask the client to put something in writing.
- Never blame other members of staff.

Reproduced with permission from Veterinary Defence Society Ltd (2003).

In addition to these general guidelines, the medical literature suggests that several factors should be taken into consideration when a veterinary practitioner is faced with a medical error (Duclos et al. 2005; Fein et al. 2007; Forster et al. 2002; Gallagher et al. 2003; Liang 2002; Mazor et al. 2004; Rosner et al. 2000):

- Clients should be made aware of all harmful errors that occur. An explicit statement that an error occurred should be conveyed in a caring, concerned and respectful manner. The disclosure should be clear, accurate, complete and non-evasive.
- An objective description of what happened, why and how, should be provided, using relationship-centred communication tools (e.g. empathy, active listening and summarizing). Clients should be allowed the opportunity to ask questions, but the vet must ensure that they do not have to 'search' for answers.
- Clients should be advised as to how, as a result of the error, lessons have been learned and how such an error can be prevented from happening in the future.
- Clients should be reassured that their case will be managed until a resolution, that is satisfactory to them, has been achieved.

Clients should, where appropriate, not incur financial liabilities because of the error. They should not, in general, be billed for veterinary fees related to the harm.

Another vital part of dealing with medical errors is the apology. Clients should receive an apology, one which conveys genuine remorse and acknowledges any upset they have experienced. (See 'What works best to dissipate anger?' earlier in this chapter.) According to Bonvicini et al. (2009), there are two types of apology: one of sympathy (e.g. 'I'm sorry that this has happened to you') and one of responsibility (e.g. 'I'm sorry that this error has happened and for the problems it has caused to you and your pet'). Evidence from human medicine suggests that patients can discriminate between the two. One review of the literature (Mazor et al. 2004) concludes that where a breach in the standard of medical care had caused harm, those patients that had received full disclosure with an apology of responsibility reported more trust and satisfaction in their doctor. A caveat to this is that, where such an adverse event occurs, it is wise to check with your professional indemnity insurers before offering such an apology, as they may require the use of a certain form of words. In instances where an animal or client has had a problem that has not resulted from medical error, an apology of sympathy is appropriate (Bonvicini et al. 2009).

Finally, it is also important to investigate the effects of mistakes on the veterinary practitioner. Making mistakes affects health care providers unfavourably (Bonvicini et al. 2009; Newman 1996), and research has shown that they can experience feelings of guilt, anxiety, disappointment or physical problems such as sleeplessness and difficulty concentrating, as a result (Gallagher et al. 2003; Mellanby & Herrtage 2004). Some even consider moving job or changing career (Mellanby & Herrtage 2004). Mellanby and Herrtage said that the impact of mistakes on the recent graduates in their study was 'often considerable, with many respondents describing feeling depressed and suffering from low self-esteem following a mistake'.

Thus, it is important that vets, following a mistake, attend to self-care or actively seek support, as well as review their case management and clinical skills (Newman 1996; Wu 2000). Finally, another way of decreasing the effects of blame on the individual is to adopt a 'systems approach', rather than a 'human approach' to human fallibility. Under the systems approach, a mistake is seen as a failure of the system, not of a person; humans are seen as fallible and errors are to be expected (Reason 2000). According to Reason (2000), 'When an adverse event occurs the important issue is not who blundered, but how and why the defences failed'.

REFERENCES

Adams CL, Bonnett BN, Meek AH (1999) Owner response to companion animal death: development of a theory and practical implication. *Canadian Veterinary Journal* 40:33–39.

Adams CL, Bonnett BN, Meek AH (2000) Predictors of owner response to companion animal death in 177 clients from 14 practices in Ontario. *Journal of the American Veterinary Medical Association* 217(9):1303–1309.

American Veterinary Medical Association (2005) AVMA Guidelines for Pet Loss Support Service. Available online: http://www.avma.org/issues/policy/pet_loss.asp (accessed 4 September 2008).

Amiel GE, Ungar L, Alperin M, Baharir Z, Cohen R, Reis S (2006) Ability of a primary care physicians to break bad news: a performance based assessment of an educational intervention. *Patient Education and Counselling* 60:10–15.

Anon (2007) Animal law expert calls for mandatory reporting of suspected animal abuse. *Veterinary Record* 161:836.

Babcock S, Neihsl A (2006) Requirements for mandatory reporting of animal cruelty. *Journal of the American Veterinary Medical Association* 228:685–689.

Benbasset J, Pilpel D, Tidhar M (1998) Patients' preferences for participation in clinical decision making. *Behavioural Medicine* 42(2):81–94.

Billson A, Tyrrell J (2003) How to break bad news. *Current Paediatrics* 13:284–287.

Bonvicini KA, O'Connell D, Cornell KK (2009) Disclosing medical errors: restoring client trust. *Compendium Continuing Education for Veterinarians* 31(3):105–112.

Brackenridge SS, Shoemaker RS (1996) The human/horse bond and client bereavement in equine practice, part 1. *Equine Practice* 18:19–23.

Bradley DW, Gehlbach SH (1988) Effect of prepaid health plans on a family practice residency. *Journal of Medical Education* 63(8):611–616.

Brown JP, Silverman JD (1999) The current and future market for veterinarians and veterinary medical services in the United States. *Journal of the American Veterinary Medical Association* 216:161–183.

Casarett D, Kutner JS, Abrahm J (for the End-of-Life Care Consensus Panel) (2001) Life after death: a practical approach to grief and bereavement. *Annals of Internal Medicine* 134(3):208–215.

Coe JB, Adams CL, Bonnett BN (2007) A focus group study of veterinarians' and pet owners' perceptions of the monetary aspects of veterinary care. *Journal of the American Veterinary Medical Association* 231(10):1510–1518.

Coulehan JL, Platt FW, Egener B, Frankel R, Lin CT, Lown B, Salazar WH (2001) 'Let me see if I have this right': words that can help build empathy. *Annals of Internal Medicine* 135:221–227.

Curtis JR, Patrick DL (1997) Barriers to communication about end-of-life care in AIDS patients. *Journal of General Internal Medicine* 12(12):736–741.

Duclos CW, Eichler M, Taylor L (2005) Patient perspectives of patient-provider communication after adverse events. *International Journal for Quality in Health Care* 17(6):479–486.

Egan G (1975) *The Skilled Helper: A Model for Systematic Helping and Interpersonal Relating*. Brooks Cole, Monterey, CA.

Epstein RM, Campbell TL, Cohen-Cole SA, McWhinney IR, Smilkstein G (1993) Perspectives on patient-doctor communication. *Journal of Family Practice* 37:377–388.

Fein SP, Hilborne LH, Spiritus EM (2007) The many faces of error disclosure: a common set of elements and a definition. *Journal of General Internal Medicine* 22:755–761.

Forster HP, Schwarz J, DeRenzo E (2002) Reducing legal risk by practicing patient-centred medicine. *Archives in Internal Medicine* 162:1217–1219.

Gallagher TH, Waterman AD, Ebers AG, Fraser VJ, Levinson W (2003) Patients' and physicians' attitudes regarding the disclosure of medical errors. *JAMA* 289(8):1001–1007.

Girgis A, Sanson-Fisher RW (1998) Breaking bad news 1: current best advice for clinicians. *Behavioral Medicine* 24(2):53–59.

GMB (2007) UK Pay League. Available online: http://www.gmb.org.uk/Templates/PressItems.asp?NodeID=96372 (accessed 14 September 2008).

Griffiths C, Foster G, Ramsay J, Eldridge S, Taylor S (2007) How effective are expert patient (lay led) programmes for chronic disease? *British Medical Journal* 334:1254–1256.

Hart L, Hart B (1987) Grief and stress from so many animal deaths. *Companion Animal Practice* 1:20–21.

Hart L, Hart BL, Mader B (1990) Humane euthanasia and companion animal death: caring for the animal, the client and the veterinarian. *Journal of the American Veterinary Medical Association* 197(10):1292–1299.

Hingorani M, Wong T, Vafidis G (1999) Patients' and doctors' attitudes to amount of information given after unintended injury during treatment: cross sectional, questionnaire survey. *British Medical Journal* 318:640–641.

Jackson JL, Kroenke K (1999) Difficult patient encounters in the ambulatory clinic: clinical predictors and outcomes. *Archives in Internal Medicine* 159:1069–1075.

Jackson JL, Kroenke K (2001) The effect of unmet expectations among adults presenting with physical symptoms. *Annals of Internal Medicine* 134:889–897.

Klingborg DJ, Klingborg J (2007) Talking with veterinary clients about money. *Veterinary Clinics of North America: Small Animal Practice* 37:79–93.

Lagoni L, Butler C, Hetts S (1994) The Human–Animal Bond and Grief. Saunders Colorado State University, Fort Collins, CO, pp. 144, 151, 172, 201, 203, 209.

Larson DG, Tobin DR (2000) End-of-life conversations. Evolving practice and theory. *JAMA* 284(12):1573–1578.

Lazoritz S (2004) Dealing with angry patients. *The Physician Executive* May–June, 28–31.

Liang BA (2002) A system of medical error disclosure. *Quality and Safety in Health Care* 11: 64–68.

Lowden B (1998) The health consequences of disclosing bad news. *European Journal of Oncology Nursing* 2(4):225–230.

Main DCJ (2006) Offering the best to patients: ethical issues associated with the provision of veterinary services. *Veterinary Record* 158:62–66.

Martin F, Ruby KL, Deking TM, Taunton AE (2004) Factors associated with client, staff, and student satisfaction regarding small animal euthanasia procedures at a veterinary teaching hospital. *Journal of the American Veterinary Medical Association* 224(11):1774–1779.

Mazor KM, Simon SR, Gurwitz JH (2004) Communicating with patients about medical errors: a review of the literature. *Archives of Internal Medicine* 164:1690–1697.

McCord RS, Floyd MR, Lang F, Young VK (2002). Responding effectively to patient anger directed at the physician. *Family Medicine* 34(5):331–336.

Mellanby RJ, Herrtage ME (2004) Survey of mistakes made by recent veterinary graduates. *Veterinary Record* 155:761–765.

Milani M (2003) Practical bond considerations: acknowledging clients' financial limits. *Canadian Veterinary Journal* 44:996–999.

Montgomery DJ (2001) Views on insurance and veterinary economics: author's response. *Journal of the American Veterinary Medical Association* 218(2):194.

Morgan CA, McDonald M (2007) Ethical dilemmas in veterinary medicine. *Veterinary Clinics of North America: Small Animal Practice* 37:165–179.

Munro HMC, Thrusfield MV (2001) Battered pets: features that raise suspicion of non-accidental injury. *Journal of Small Animal Practice* 42:218–226.

Newman M (1996) The emotional impact of mistakes on family physicians. *Archives of Family Medicine* 5(2):71.

O'Connell D, Bonvicini KA (2007) Addressing disappointment in veterinary practice. *Vet Clinics of North America: Small Animal Practice* 37(1):135–149.

Osborne CA (2001) What are veterinarians worth? *Journal of the American Veterinary Medical Association* 219(3):302–303.

Osborne CA (2002) Client confidence in veterinarians: how can it be sustained? *Journal of the American Veterinary Medical Association* 221(7):936–938.

Persaud R (2007) Questioning 'culture of death': why are vets prone to suicide? *Veterinary Times* November 19, pp. 6–7.

Platt FW, Keller VF (1994) Empathic communication: a teachable and learnable skill. *Journal of General Internal Medicine* 9:222–226.

Ptacek JT, Ptacek JJ (2001) Patients' perceptions of receiving bad news about cancer. *Journal of Clinical Oncology* 19(2):4160–4164.

Reason J (2000) Human error: models and management. *British Medical Journal* 320:768–770.

Roen DT (2001) Views on insurance and veterinary economics. *Journal of the American Veterinary Medical Association* 218(2):194.

Rosner F, Berger JT, Kark P, Potash J, Bennett AJ (2000) Disclosure and prevention of medical errors. *Archives in Internal Medicine* 160:2089–2092.

Royal College of Veterinary Surgeons (2008) *Guide to Professional Conduct.* RCVS, London.

Schmid Mast M, Kindlimann A, Langewitz W (2005) Recipients' perspective on breaking bad news: how you put it really makes a difference. *Patient Education and Counselling* 58:244–251.

Shaw J, Baker M (2004) Expert patient – dream or nightmare? *British Medical Journal* 328:723–724.

Shaw JR, Lagoni L (2007) End-of-life communication in veterinary medicine: delivering bad news and euthanasia decision making. *Veterinary Clinics of North America: Small Animal Practice* 37:95–108.

Short D (1994) Learning from our mistakes. *British Journal of Hospital Medicine* 51:250–252.

Silverman J, Kurtz S, Draper J (2005) *Skills for Communicating with Patients*, 2nd edn. Radcliffe Medical, Oxford.

Slater MR, Barton CL, Rogers KS, Peterson JL, Harris C, Wallace K (1996) Factors affecting treatment decisions and satisfaction of owners of cats with cancer. *Journal of the American Veterinary Medical Association* 208:1248–1252.

Tarn DM, Paterniti DA, Heritage J (2006) Physician communication about the cost and acquisition of newly prescribed medications. *American Journal of Managed Care* 12(11):657–664.

Tinga CE, Adams CL, Bonnett BN, Ribble CS (2001) Survey of veterinary technical and professional skills in students and recent graduates of a veterinary college. *Journal of the American Veterinary Medical Association* 219(7):924–931.

Tulsky JA (2005) Beyond advance directives: importance of communication skills at the end of life. *Journal of the American Medical Association* 294(3):359–366.

Veterinary Defence Society Ltd (2003) *The VDS: Complaints and How to Deal with Them – A Guide for Veterinary Practices.* The Veterinary Defence Society, Knutsford, Cheshire.

Vincent C, Philips A, Young M (1994) Why do people sue doctors? A study of patients and relatives taking legal action. *Lancet* 343(8913):1609–1613.

von Gunten CF, Ferris FD, Emanuel LL (2000) Ensuring competency in end-of-life care: communication and relational skills. *JAMA* 284(23):3051–3057.

Waldsmith JK (2003) Horse owner education for practice development: financial benefits of horse owner education. Paper presented at 49th Annual Convention of the American Association of Equine Practitioners, 2003, New Orleans, LA.

Wasan AD, Wootton J, Jamison RN (2005) Dealing with difficult patients in your pain practice. *Regional Anaesthesia and Pain Medicine* 30(2):184–192.

Weingart SN, McL Wilson R, Gibberd RW, Harrison, B (2000) Epidemiology of medical error. *British Medical Journal* 320:774–777.

Weissman DE (2004) Decision making at a time of crisis near the end of life. *JAMA* 292(14):1738–1744.

Wensley SP (2008) Animal welfare and the human-animal bond: considerations for veterinary faculty, students, and practitioners. *Journal Veterinary Medical Education* 35(4):532–539.

Whitford RE (2004) Future prosperity depends on consumer trust. *Journal of the American Veterinary Medical Association* 225(12):1824–1825.

Wojciechowska J, Hewson CJ (2005) Quality-of-life assessment in pet dogs. *Journal of the American Veterinary Medical Association* 226(5):722–728.

Wu AW (2000) Medical error: the second victim. *British Medical Journal* 320:726–727.

Communicating with colleagues

6

Geoff Little

Introduction

'No man is an island' (Donne 1624), and when it comes to veterinary practices, even those that are designated 'single-handed' are not really true to the strict definition. Even the smallest practice will comprise more than one individual, and once there is more than one, communication, or lack of it, becomes an issue.

One would think that in a relatively small enterprise the presence of good communication could be taken for granted. After all, how difficult can it be to ensure that a small number of individuals, working as a team, in a relatively small area, know exactly what the objectives of that business are, what policies are in place and what each individual's role is in making it happen?

Let us not assume for a minute that the practising arm of our profession is unique in having a problem in communicating with colleagues, but it does seem to be an all too often finding by those who are called in to review the business side of practices, and we know that poor communication can lead to niggles, complaints and in extremis to claims of negligence or misconduct.

The word 'communication' comes from the Latin *communicare* meaning to impart, to share or to make common. As the word suggests, it is not a one-way event, and communication needs to flow in all directions to ensure the smooth running of an effective and efficient business. It is said that in 'face-to-face' communication, the words account for only 7% of what is conveyed, the rest being through body language and tone of voice. When it comes to communicating with colleagues, either in the same practice or between practices, words may be important, but how we treat colleagues in terms of our attitude and our body language is just as important.

In this chapter, we look at some of the ways in which communication between colleagues can be improved for the benefit of all, including our clients and our patients. We shall address

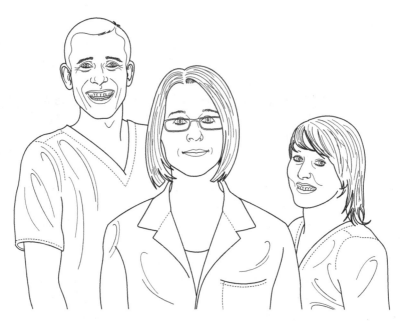

Figure 6.1   Every team deserves a good leader.

the subject of intrapractice communication as it affects the practice in isolation, as well as the ever-increasing challenge of interpractice communication as more and more practices network over referrals and out-of-hours emergency work.

THE TEAM AND ITS LEADER

Every team deserves a good leader (Figure 6.1) who has the vision to see where they want to take their business, the confidence to know that the destination they are heading towards is the correct one, and the wisdom to know when, along that journey, adjustments need to be made to alter course. Leaders must have the ability to communicate that vision to the team as a whole and must know its constituent members well enough to understand what motivates each and every one of them, thereby ensuring everybody's efforts are channelled in the same direction, and that as a result the destination is reached with as many of the team on board as possible. In reality, the destination should be a rolling horizon, with the business constantly looking at where it is heading. Although it is said that the enjoyment is all too often in the travelling rather than in the destination, nothing motivates like success and it certainly pays to have specific milestones along every trip, where one can rest briefly and celebrate the achievement, before setting off on the journey again.

What constitutes good leadership in today's veterinary practice is no different from what succeeds in other business sectors. Most veterinary practices are small in terms of personnel numbers, dictating a flat management structure, which encourages flexibility, innovation and commitment rather than the more traditional hierarchical structure found in larger businesses, which is now somewhat out of fashion and which relied on command and control, adherence to strictly laid down procedures, with clear and narrow responsibilities. This latter method of managing teams is probably best represented in the armed forces where it still has a place, but in today's veterinary practices, the more successful ones are empowering team members and delegating areas of responsibilities to them.

When team members are asked what is important to them in their job, the following responses will usually appear high on the list of responses:

- Confidence in the leader
- A sense of belonging
- Excitement in the job

Although 'confidence in the team leader' may be something team members express, it is a reflected opinion and more than likely the result of that leader behaving in a specific way. If one were to ask why that confidence exists, it would probably be because that leader possessed some or all of the following attributes:

- Vision
- Enthusiasm
- Adaptability
- Integrity
- Toughness
- Fairness
- Warmth
- Humility
- Confidence

That is quite a shopping list, and at first glance some of the attributes may appear to be contradictory. For example, how can one exhibit warmth and toughness at the same time? How can one be confident and at the same time be humble? The answer lies in two of the other attributes on the list, fairness and adaptability. Abraham Maslow, the American psychologist, said, 'When the only tool you have is a hammer, all problems tend to resemble nails' (Maslow 1966).

The effective leader will have a comprehensive toolbox and will know just when to reach for a different tool, when to apply it, and will know just the correct amount of strength and/or leverage to apply to get the job done.

This is not a book about leadership as such, but the role the leader plays is so important and has a major part to play in the success or otherwise of the team. Everything the leader does communicates something to the team, and so it is totally justifiable and appropriate to spend a little more time considering the role of the leader.

In considering the list of traits required to lead a team, some may be in-built features of an individual's personality, whereas others may have to be learnt and/or developed. The leader should lead by example, but all too often when it comes to adhering to standard operating procedures (SOPs) in a practice, the main culprit or culprits are those who the rest of the team should be looking to for example. If the boss flouts the rules, then it must be okay for the rest of the team to do likewise.

Types of people

If we exclude start-ups, practice teams are established units, comprising individuals functioning at varying levels of effectiveness and efficiency. A good deal of research has been carried out into the types of people that make up teams, including the ways in which they communicate with each other.

There is a whole industry out there, employing various methods of analysing individuals, seeking to categorize and label them according to their responses to questionnaires. And once labelled, these individuals are expected to respond in certain ways to differing sets of circumstances and because of that to contribute to teams in different ways. For example, some individuals may exhibit leadership skills, other will be the ideas people and yet others will be the ones at the sharp end dutifully following SOPs. Reading the horoscope pages in some publications, one could be excused for thinking that the predictions for individuals born under the star sign Taurus read remarkably like the forecasts for those born under the star sign Scorpio, or indeed for those born under any of the other ten star signs. However, the traits for the different types, as defined by the Belbin, Myers-Briggs or other industry-standard typology methods (see suggestions for further reading), are sufficiently diverse, recognized and repeated in individuals to lend credibility to the belief that people can be categorized and that within those categories individuals will behave in certain ways.

Why should this be of interest to veterinary practices? Well, as has already been mentioned, practices are teams, however small that team may be, and the success or otherwise of each team will depend on, not only the individual skills within the team, but how the team functions as a cohesive unit. A good team will produce results, which are consistently better than the expected sum of the abilities of the individuals within that team.

Replacing and/or recruiting new team members

The introduction of a new practice member is a golden opportunity to introduce new skills into the team or to strengthen existing ones. Too many practices spend too little time on maximizing this opportunity. All too often like is replaced with like; self-clones are appointed or 'the best of a bad lot' is selected.

In taking on a new employee, there are responsibilities on both sides. There is a responsibility to new appointees in terms of doing everything possible to ensure their success in the team. The mature employee will probably be leaving another post in the hope of bettering themselves, while the first-time employee is at a vulnerable point in their career and needs a supportive environment in which to develop. In both cases, the onus is on the employer to facilitate a smooth integration into the existing team for the sake of the individual, the team and the business.

Communication with new employees starts at the advertising stage. The advertisement needs to impart enough information to appeal to a sufficient number of suitable individuals to provide the employer with a large enough pool from which to choose their new team member(s). Reference has already been made to 'employing the best of a bad lot', and sometimes this is the fault of the advertisement in as much as it has not provided sufficient, accurate information. As practice teams increase in terms of numbers, roles become more specialized and as a result employers need to be more specific in terms of the search criteria they include in their advertisements. For example, if a practice needs to recruit a receptionist, the advertisement should make it clear that this role involves working with people as opposed to with animals. All too often, the word 'veterinary' in an advertisement conveys the prospect of working with animals to those reading it.

One of the most common complaints from recent graduates is that promises made at interviews have not been kept. Promises of regular practice meetings, appraisals, personal development plans and support during the first few weeks in a new practice are regularly cited as being mentioned during the interview but never materializing. It would appear that employers know what is wanted by new graduates and so they know what noises to make at the interview but, for a variety of reasons, fail to deliver. The interview is an important opportunity for both sides to communicate just what is on offer from the practice and what the potential new recruit wants. The written word, in the form of the job advertisement, on the one side, and the application letter and the CV, on the other, can communicate only so much. The face-to-face meeting allows the gaps to be filled and provides the opportunity to probe deeper into what has been written. From the prospective employee's point of view, they need to know not only all the details of the job on offer but get a feel for the practice and the culture in place. Interviewees should attend the interview with a clear picture of what they need to know about the job on offer. They should go armed with a list of questions they want to have the answers to and should not be afraid to refer to the list during the interview, to double check all areas have been covered. At the end of the formal interview, both sides should have a clear picture of the position on offer and the suitability of the candidate to fill that role. The interviewee should leave with a copy of the job description and the terms of employment.

As the new recruit will be joining the rest of the team, it makes sense to extend the formal interview into an opportunity for the rest of the team to meet and provide feedback on the perceived suitability of the potential new member. Spending some informal time in the practice, with other team members, will also provide the interviewee with the opportunity to talk to the colleagues they may subsequently be working with.

INDUCTION SCHEMES AND MENTORING

A new member of the team can feel very isolated, in particular recent veterinary graduates who will have come from a very supportive network of friends at university and at home. In the majority of cases, it will be the first time they have been away from direct, structured support, and despite modern communications, they often perceive themselves as isolated, having to cope with a whole new set of circumstances and associated challenges. A supportive practice may well have structures in place such as a set of SOPs, which the new team member can refer to and will hopefully offer direct support, should the new graduate have to cope with out-of-hours calls, but having a structured induction scheme and appointing a mentor to look after new recruits can provide so much more for the benefit of all concerned.

It would serve all those who own and run their own practices to recall just what it was like during those initial few days and weeks in their first job; how different it was to be the one who now had responsibilities to clients and other team members as opposed to one's previous role perhaps as an undergraduate undertaking EMS (extramural studies) and having somebody else to take those ultimate decisions.

It would also serve those who own veterinary businesses to remember that they are placing new recruits in front of and amongst the two most valuable assets they have. No, it is not the colour Doppler machine or the new digital X-ray machine. These assets per se do not even appear on the balance sheet. What are they? The first is the client base and the second is the practice team members. Without either, there is no business. All too often though, new recruits, whose only prior contact with the practice may have been at a relatively short interview, are let loose in the practice with the assumption that they either have what it takes or that they will pick things up as they go along. And when it comes to the latter attitude, all too often the problem can be compounded by allowing those new recruits to learn from others who themselves have picked things up in a haphazard way.

It is far better to take stock of just what it says in the new recruit's job description, what their CV tells you about their level of experience, where they will be working in the practice, what their tasks will include and who they will be working with. If all that is taken into account, an induction programme can be devised which, depending on their role in the practice, may include the shadowing of different people in the practice, for varying periods. The aim of this initial investment in new team members should be not only to provide them with adequate knowledge of the business's services, products and working practices, but it should also instil in them enough insight to allow them to promote the business with confidence.

APPRAISALS

There are certain words or phrases that seem to elicit a less than positive response, 'appraisals' being one of them and 'mission statement' another. If, on the other hand, instead of an appraisal we were to speak about a structured process that has two main objectives: the first to develop the individual within the team and the second to improve the effectiveness of that team, I believe the majority of individuals would buy into it. Just do not call the process an appraisal. Similarly, if the practice team were tasked with drawing up a list of what they wanted the practice to achieve when it came to patients and clients in terms of the service provided and the practice itself where working conditions were concerned, there would not be too many objections. Just do not call the list a mission statement.

Let us start by looking at the downside of carrying out appraisals. Done well, they are time-consuming as they need to be carried out on a regular basis, say, every 6 months; a great deal of thought and preparation needs to be given to the structure, process and the content of each appraisal, and in the ideal world everybody in the team, including the bosses, should be appraised.

Because most employees either will have had first-hand experience of or will have preconceived ideas of appraisals, it is best to introduce the concept at a full practice meeting. In that way, the benefits can be extolled and fears can be allayed.

The process itself is fairly straightforward and comprises the following steps:

1. The appraiser completes an appraisal form for each team member.
2. The appraisee completes a similar form.
3. At the appraisal meeting, the contents of the two forms are discussed and compared.
4. By the end of the meeting, a way forward is agreed and a date is set for the next appraisal.

Bearing in mind the *raison d'être* is to help to develop the individual, vital elements of the process are for the appraiser to have a clear understanding as to both the appraisee's job description and how well that team member has performed against criteria agreed at the last appraisal.

The forms facilitate the process as both the appraiser and the appraisee complete these prior to the meeting. The forms cover the activities of the individual, their responsibilities and their aspirations, and sufficient time must be allowed for both sides to consider their responses. Although there will be a general theme where the forms are concerned, there will be a need to compile different appraisal forms to suit the varying practice roles. The completed forms can be contrasted and compared at the appraisal meeting, the outcome of which should be the following:

- A consensus as to how well the individual is performing
- A reassessment as to the individual's role and responsibilities within the team and a re-alignment if necessary
- An agreed way forward and, where appropriate, a setting of SMART objectives, meaning:
  ○ Specific
  ○ Measurable
  ○ Achievable
  ○ Realistic
  ○ Timed – a date in the diary for the next appraisal

Appraisals are part of the way of life in large businesses and, believe it or not, young employees in those organizations look forward to their appraisals. They regard the process as positive in that it is the time they receive positive feedback on how they have performed since their last appraisal. In addition, at the end of the meeting new goals are set for them to attain and a plan is put in place to provide them with the necessary support and training to reach those goals. It is all part of the vital task of developing the person who in turn will develop your practice. And remember, if you do not develop your people, the good ones will find somebody else who will.

EXIT INTERVIEW

When it comes to the employer–employee relationship, the exit interview completes the circle. The employment interview is an opportunity to find out more about the interviewee and to fill the gaps between the lines on the CV. It is also the time to inform the prospective new team member about your practice. The exit interview reverses those roles in as much as it provides the opportunity for the soon to be ex-team member to tell you about your business and you an individual. Inevitably, individuals leave practices and one should not miss the opportunity to benefit from those individuals' insights into the team and the way the practice is run from their perspective and those they work with. Irrespective of how good communications are within a practice, groups develop with barriers between them. In well-run practices where communications are good, those barriers are low and porous and information flows between the groups, but in badly run practices those barriers are insurmountable, and whereas information fails to breach the barriers, misinformation seems to have little difficulty in filtering through. To compound the problem, communication within each group appears to function well, allowing rumours to flourish, resulting in an entrenchment of views and ever-rising barriers.

In the exit interview, it is important to have an objective, depersonalized, constructive discussion with the individual who is leaving. From the employer's perspective, the object of the exercise is to gain information from the departing employee that will prove useful to improve the ongoing business. They may shed light on how the practice could be improved in terms of the service to clients or on what changes could be introduced to improve the working conditions, which, in turn, could lead to a more contented and cohesive team, and would almost inevitably have the knock-on effect of providing a better service to clients and patients alike, a win, win, win situation.

DELEGATION

One of the key objectives of any practice owner, leader or manager is to achieve their goals through the efforts of others (Figure 6.2). There may well be differences between individuals in terms of qualifications and abilities, but the one thing we all have an equal amount of is 'hours in the day'.

Unfortunately, all too often it is a case of abdication rather than delegation with team members being left to get on with it with little or no instructions or backup. The other major fault is too much interference having delegated the task, with bosses leaning over the shoulders of others, pointing out how they would have done things. The result is an undermining of confidence, an attitude of, 'Why don't you do it yourself?' and a reluctance to volunteer to take on further tasks.

To achieve our objectives we have to motivate and delegate to others. The basic components of successful delegation are as follows:

1. Communicate to the individual(s) what it is you want them to do. If it is a specific task, make it SMART or ideally SMARTER. (See p 135)
2. Provide the necessary support in terms of materials and training and advice.
3. Monitor progress without interfering.
4. Encourage feedback and continue to offer support.

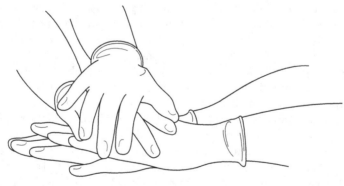

Figure 6.2   Motivation.

otivation

ow does one create a motivated workforce? What can you do to motivate others? One way answer this question is to look at the end result. In other words, what does a motivated terinary practice look like and how does it behave? What would you see and experience you were a client or a potential new employee and were to walk into such a practice? As a ent, you would see people enjoying their work, individuals who are knowledgeable and ho, although they may not know the answer to all the questions, do know where to go or hom to ask in order to find out, personnel who take pride in the place they work and who ep their promises.

What would it be like to work alongside such motivated individuals? You would see ergetic and enthusiastic individuals working well together as a team, focused on achieving sults and celebrating success, team members who avoid blaming others when difficulties ise but who look to find solutions to problems.

In looking for the answers to what we can do to motivate others and to create a team that nctions as described above, it pays to take time out to ask ourselves who or what motivates . In other words, what gets us out of bed in the morning?

The reality is that different things motivate different individuals and different things mo- ate the same individual at different times during their life and career. All too often, we sume that money is the prime motivator of others, whereas as long as the financial remu- ration is fair for the role being undertaken, the prime motivators are intrinsic rather than trinsic and include such things as:

Having an interesting job
Working within a fair environment
Having goals to strive for
Receiving recognition and being regarded as an important member of the team

Extrinsic factors such as financial bonuses can play a role in motivating individuals and ams but do need to be used with care. It must always be borne in mind that every action n have an opposite and not always equal reaction. Rewarding one individual financially ay incentivize that person but may well demotivate all the other team members, and the e incentivized member may require ever-increasing rewards to keep them motivated. If e wants to use money as a motivator, it should be done with caution. To be meaningful, a ancial bonus needs to be of a reasonable magnitude compared with the basic salary. The teria on which the bonus is paid, or not, as the case may be, need to be simple, transparent d under the direct control of the individual or individuals the incentive applies to. They ed to be SMART and a great deal of consideration needs to be given to those criteria, as e consequences to both the individual and the business of the bonus not being paid must considered.

TANDARD OPERATING PROCEDURES

mmunication comes in many forms, and when there is a need to disseminate important ormation, for example, statutory matters such as ionizing radiation regulations, man- l handling operations, special waste regulations and the host of other health and safety

SMARTER Objectives

The term SMART Objectives is originally attributed to Peter Drucker; it appeared
management book, *The Practice of Management*, with the acronym usually standir

Specific
Measurable
Achievable
Realistic
Time-bound

There have been many variations on the original theme, some of which are as

S	Stimulating	Simple			
M	Motivating				
A	Appropriate	Attainable	Accepted	Accountable	Agreed A
R	Relevant				
T	Timed	Trackable	Traceable		

It is understandable that the original SMART acronym tends to follow the think
1950s in as much as it has that slight dictatorial note to it, and one can imagine th
objective being imposed from on high, without too much discussion with those wh
instructed to carry out the task.

Looking at some of the alternatives to the letters above, such as 'accepted' and
one can see the transition to a more modern approach to managing teams, more
nication and a greater involvement of team members. The acronym SMARTER in
the new words, 'extending' and 'rewarding', which highlight the importance of e
individuals. SMARTER objectives can also be employed in agreeing and setting the
development goals for team members. Provided that adequate support is in place,
ing individuals for their achievements in coping with, and hopefully excelling at, ex
tasks is a very powerful motivational force.

A management objective to increase the number of appointments being booke
receptionists is not a SMART objective. Neither is a plan to introduce a nurse-run se
clinic into the practice some time during the current year. The following, however,
classed as SMART management objectives:

From 3 months' time, a minimum of 85% of available appointment slots will be
when averaged over the calendar week.

Within 6 months, the nursing team will have planned and conducted two senio
clinics and one such clinic will be run each month thereafter.

When introducing new ideas into a practice, it is much better to target easy win
There is nothing like success to motivate individuals and the team to move on to the r
more ambitious task.

regulations a practice has to deal with, clear, relevant information in a written format is best suited to the job.

Written SOPs are also the best medium when it comes to ensuring team members adhere to agreed methods when carrying out specific, frequently occurring procedures in the practice. SOPs can cover such diverse topics as registering new clients, credit policy, admitting and discharging patients, etc.

In essence, an SOP should provide detailed written instructions to achieve uniformity of the performance of a specific function. When it comes to producing an SOP, it is advisable to ask those most involved in the process to have the first stab at producing a draft. All too often SOPs are produced and imposed by management who may not have first-hand knowledge of the situation, resulting in a list of instructions to be followed that are impractical. It is hardly surprising that team members fail to follow the protocol.

Far better, for example, to ask the kennel hand to write the SOP for cleaning the kennel area or the feeding of in-patients, but only after they have been given advice and training on how to write an SOP. In its simplest form an SOP should have a title; the person writing it should *write down what they do* and those who are involved in that process should *do what is written down*. It is as simple as that. The aim is to have a written procedure that is agreed and utilized. It should be written in terms that are easily understood by all. Some SOPs are best written as narratives, others as flowcharts or tables. The draft document should be circulated throughout the team and comments are sought before the final SOP is adopted.

If one considers why SOPs fail in the workplace, we can take steps to ensure their usage. Common reasons are as follows:

- They are difficult to find.
- They are written in a 'foreign language'.
- Instructions and general information are mixed.
- The procedure is described in an unfamiliar way.
- Users know a better method and can do the procedure 'in their sleep'.

Senior members of the team often fall into the category of those 'who know a better method' – after all they have been doing it their way for years and SOPs are for the staff, not for them. When it comes to SOPs it is very important to lead by example. If you do not, it will hardly be surprising if others take short cuts too, sometimes with disastrous results.

It is best to aim to end up with the SOP on one side of A4 and in large font. Stick to simple words and short sentences. Think the process through in your mind and capture the procedure in a list of instructions, 'Do this', 'Do that'. Make sure the list is in the correct order and separate instructions from information. Incorporate diagrams or tables, but only if it helps to simplify and clarify the SOP. Provide references at the end. These may include a reference to another SOP.

SOPs should be regarded as living documents, ones that the team become familiar with, but beware the danger of familiarity breeding complacency. SOPs should be either displayed in a prominent area or easily accessed in, for example, a folder or on the practice intranet. Having them on the intranet not only allows easy access but facilitates amendments, which should be carried out as and when needs arise. Another common reason why team members fail to adhere to SOPs is that as time moves on, new medicines become available, new equipment is introduced and the existing SOP becomes outdated. When it is discovered that a number of team members are not adhering to an SOP, it may not be them that need looking at but the SOP.

As time evolves, the number of SOPs in use will inevitably increase and most practices find themselves with a 'Practice Bible' to house all the paperwork that can be issued to all team members to read, inwardly digest and to use for reference. The 'Practice Bible' also serves as a useful publication to issue to new employees as part of their induction. Some practices find it useful to ask new recruits to sign a declaration that they have read and understood the contents; some practices, in the belief that it is all too easy to sign to say you have done something, put new team members through a brief test to ensure they have read and fully understood the contents.

Box 6.1 shows an example of an SOP for euthanasia, setting out easy-to-read, clear instructions, for all team members to follow.

Box 6.1   A standard operating procedure for euthanasia

Euthanasia is considered by many to be the most important procedure that we are asked to carry out as veterinarians. It is a very emotive time for clients and where possible such consultations should be booked in at a time when sufficient, quality time can be devoted to the procedure. It is a procedure that must never be hurried.

The euthanasia procedure must be discussed with the client before any action is carried out. The veterinarian should inform the client that there might be some post-mortem muscular spasms, 'reflex breathing', and that their pet's eyes may remain open.

The owner should be given the option to be present or not when the procedure is carried out. If they decide not to remain with their pet, they should be given the option to see their pet afterwards.

Disposal

Before euthanasia is carried out, the disposal of the body is to be discussed with the owner or their agent. The following options are to be offered:

- Home burial
- General cremation
- Private cremation
- Burial at the pet cemetery

Cremation or commercial burial

If the client opts for cremation or burial, all options, with associated costs, should be discussed with them. Their decision should be recorded on the patient's clinical records and the appropriate paperwork should be completed.

Consent form

Go through the Euthanasia Consent Form and ensure that the client or the client's agent signs the form before the procedure is carried out.

Procedure

Intravenous phenobarbitone via the cephalic vein is the procedure of choice in cats and dogs. If the owner wishes to hold their pet and it is deemed safe for them and the operators to do so, they should be permitted. The patient should be restrained by a member of support staff to facilitate the administration of the intravenous injection. Where manual restraint or muzzling is considered to be too stressful for either the pet or its owner or dangerous for the operators, a sedative may be administered to the patient prior to the intravenous injection. Where hospitalized cases have an indwelling intravenous catheter is in place, it should be used to administer the phenobarbitone.

Accidental injection

Extreme care must be taken to avoid accidental injection of personnel. If accidental injection should occur, seek medical attention immediately and record the incident in the accident book.

Hospitalized cases

Where hospitalized cases are to be euthanized, the owner or the owner's agent is to be given the option to be present when the procedure takes place. It is not necessary to insist on the client attending the practice to sign a Euthanasia Consent Form, but permission must be obtained and details of that permission must be recorded on the clinical notes.

Payment

The option of paying for the procedure in the consulting room should be given to avoid the upset of clients being embarrassed at reception. Clients may also be given the option of being sent an account if thought appropriate.

Records

Details of the euthanasia along with the chosen route of disposal must be entered onto the computer records. An appropriate tag must be completed to identify the body and the chosen method of disposal. This tag must accompany the body until it is collected from the practice. Details of the pet, its owner and the tag number must also be entered in the pet crematorium record book.

Storage

When the body has been placed in the appropriate disposal bag and labelled with the client's and pet's details, it must be placed in the freezer to await collection.

STAFF SUGGESTION SCHEME

Outside the corporate world, virtually all practice owners are self-appointed and have arrived in that position through hard work and having made decisions at various times during the life of the business. We live in a world where the rate of change is exponential, where information is coming at us from all directions and different sectors of the marketplace have differing wants and needs. Take, for example, the differing ways in which the various generations communicate, the ways in which they differ in terms of seeking and acting upon information, the ways in which they conduct business. Ten years ago, nobody would have come into a veterinary practice clutching a wad of printed information gathered from the internet in an attempt to help the veterinary surgeon to work their way through a complicated set of symptoms and laboratory results, in an attempt to clinch a diagnosis. We may not always agree with the direction in which so-called progress is taking us, but the only constant is change. The leader of any team has to be aware of what is happening in the marketplace and should be making the best use of the market intelligence that may be available under their noses, in other words, within the team members.

The list of qualities required to be a good leader are many, and established leaders will have some or all of those qualities in varying degrees. Having said that, the production of good ideas is not the sole prerogative of the leader and others in the team may well have an idea or ideas that could enhance the business, or one aspect of it. A germ of an idea may reside within any team member and at any time; it may come from a seasoned member of the team who is conversant with the way the business is currently run; it may come from a new member of the team who has brought knowledge with them gained from working in another veterinary practice, or indeed another line of work, or it may come from the most junior individual, fresh out of school, who has not yet had the flair and enthusiasm knocked out of them.

Tom Peters, author of *In Search of Excellence* (Peters & Waterman 2004) and a world-renowned business consultant, when called in to advise a board of directors that had been informed by a number of their customers that 'their products were boring', took one look at the board and told them that it was no wonder their products were boring and asked them when they had last taken a critical look at themselves as they were boring, all men in their late 50s, all dressed in dark suits, white shirts and plain dark ties. His advice to them was to bring some interesting people into the boardroom who had done something different in their lives and who came from different backgrounds. Perhaps they could do something interesting with the company's products.

From a veterinary perspective, we no longer frown on those who have taken a year off to do something else. Indeed, this may lead them to suggesting innovative ideas for change when they return to practice.

We all have greater expectations when it comes to service industries, and veterinary practice is no different. Our clients have ever-rising expectations, and practices need new ideas and better processes to ensure we continue to best look after them and the animals under our care. If practices want to flourish, they can no longer survive with team members who rely on management to come up with all the 'right answers'. Today's successful practices need to encourage all team members to come up with a steady flow of new ideas and solutions, especially from those who are most intimately involved with and are affected by the processes and from the clients, those at the sharp end. Good ideas for improving processes in the kennel room are less likely to come from the large animal partner in a mixed practice, and much more likely to come from those who spend their day in that particular part of the building.

Having good ideas is one thing, but capturing them and progressing them is another thing altogether. There needs to be a process in place to encourage the generation of good ideas. The mere existence of a structure lets the whole team know that the process of generating ideas is encouraged. The process needs to be explained to the team at a practice meeting, and although the discussion may well be far and wide ranging, the only two questions that really need to be answered are, who will benefit from it and how is it going to work?

Who will it benefit?

It must be remembered that whenever one is trying to 'sell' anything to anybody, although that product or service will have features and functions, people are seeking to buy benefits.

The features of a certain MP3 player may include 8 Gb of memory, USB connectivity, 24 hours of battery life following a full charge that takes only 90 minutes, all in an impact-resistant case with armband. All very interesting, but most people, however, will decide to purchase it because those features allow it to store up to 5500 audio tracks or 32 hours of video files, it is quick to charge and can be used all day before it needs to be recharged and the 'it comes in an impact-resistant case with armband' means it can be used in the gym and while out jogging.

Before introducing any new concept to the team or to clients ask yourself, 'Why should they be interested in it?', or 'What's in it for them?'

How will it work?

In introducing the idea of a staff suggestion scheme, it is important to follow the theme of benefits and to provide guidance as to what areas the suggestions should cover. For example, the message could go out that suggestions should be aimed at looking at the following:

- Ways of enhancing working conditions within the practice
- Ways of improving current SOPs
- Ways of enhancing the current service to clients
- New services and products that should be introduced

There needs to be a mechanism in place to capture the suggestions. Like all processes, the easier it can be made, the more likely it is to be used and the greater the uptake is likely to be.

Suggestions should be submitted on forms that are easy to complete, and which facilitate the capturing of the idea, why and how to introduce it into the practice and who will benefit from its introduction.

Once submitted, there will naturally be an air of expectation from the individual who generated the idea, and because of that there needs to be a guarantee in place that all suggestions will receive an initial response in writing within a prescribed period, say, 1 week. If the response is no, that needs to be conveyed. If it is a winner and can be introduced without further deliberation, state when it will be introduced. If it is a qualified yes, provide a date for further reply and stick to that commitment. It may well be appropriate to involve the individual or individuals who promoted the idea in a working party to move things forward. A practice would need to decide whether to make the process public when it comes to replying to suggestions, posting responses on a designated notice board or in a printed update or by electronic mail. The argument for a public response is that quite often, when one individual submits an idea, he or she is voicing what is on the minds of a number of team members and that the entire team should be included in the feedback. The argument against this is that making the process a public affair may inhibit individuals from taking part.

Another decision a practice will have to take when it comes to a suggestion scheme is whether there should be a monetary reward involved for those whose suggestions are adopted by the practice. This is common practice in big business and can take many forms. Some schemes involve a multi-step evaluation process, with those who submitted the successful ones eventually receiving either a fixed sum or one related to the anticipated value of the idea to the business.

An alternative approach would be to dedicate a fixed amount to the scheme, which is then distributed on a monthly basis, with fixed sums being awarded to the best idea or ideas each month. Once the staff know that you are serious about the scheme and they see the benefits on a monthly basis, the suggestion box should be filled with suggestions to consider. The real benefits, of course, will be seen by all team members in a better run and more enjoyable place to work.

PRACTICE MEETINGS

If you speak to individuals who carry out independent practice reviews where all members of the team are asked, amongst other things, to carry out a SWOT analysis (strengths, weaknesses, opportunities and threats) on their business, lack of communication will feature on most people's responses, along with a desire to have more practice meetings. These sentiments are repeated over and over again whenever the subject of improving practice is discussed. It is common to hear young graduates tell of unfulfilled expectations in their first job, of promises made at interview that remain mere promises 15 months later. Most employers seem to acknowledge the importance of regular practice meetings as they would appear to be a common topic of conversation at interview, but in too many instances they fail to materialize. And there are all too many excuses as to why they remain an intention rather than a reality: 'It's hard to find a time that suits, to get everybody together' or 'We've tried practice meetings, they go on forever and just end up as slanging matches and anyway nothing constructive every happens afterwards, so we stopped having them'.

Practice meetings are the most effective way of ensuring good communications within the practice at all levels, but only if they are structured to be efficient and effective.

There are a number of key decisions to take when it comes to deciding on the nature and number of practice meetings to be held. Amongst the questions that need to be answered are the following:

- Which types of meeting need to be held and what are the functions of each type?
- Who should attend each type of meeting and why?
- Which types of meeting need to be held on a regular basis, and how often?
- Is there a call for one-off meetings?

It is probably fair to say that the larger the practice, the greater the need to have regular structured meetings, but even the smallest single-handed practice may well benefit from regular meetings rather than relying on discussions held over the operating table or as and when time permits.

Types of meeting

Every business needs to be led and as such there needs to be a plan for people to follow, and those team members need to be provided with the motivation and the tools to follow that plan.

Assuming there is a business plan in place, a plan that has defined SMART objectives, meaning they are specific, measurable, achievable, realistic and timed, there will be a need to hold regular meetings to monitor progress to ensure the business is on track, and if it is not, to decide on measures to introduce to get it back on track. In a larger business this would be the equivalent of board meetings which directors and executive would attend. The equivalent in the practice would be the partners and the practice manager, and depending on where a practice is in terms of its journey, the meetings may be held monthly if it is at the start of its journey or bimonthly or even quarterly, if it is well on track.

Decisions taken at board level are then passed on to executives to implement, and it is the role of the executives and managers to ensure the plan is achieved through the efforts of the team members. Generally speaking, veterinary practices, because of smaller personnel numbers, tend to have flatter management structures than those found in bigger businesses and, as a result, do not have the numbers to allow for a vertical management structure with well-defined, singular roles.

Irrespective of the type of meeting, there are some essentials that will help to ensure their effectiveness and efficiency.

Scheduling

It is very difficult to find a time that suits everybody when it comes to fixing a date for subsequent meetings. If the last item on the agenda is 'date of next meeting', there is the inevitable fumbling for diaries to find a date when all members of the group are next free, in say, 2 months' time. There will be those who did not bring their diaries, those who brought the wrong diary and those who will have to check their partner's diary and the calendar on the kitchen wall when they get home to find a free date. It is much better to fix the dates well in advance so that these commitments can go in diaries for the foreseeable future. If the meetings are to be held bimonthly, set the dates, for example, for the second Tuesday of every other month. That way there can be no excuse for people not knowing when the meetings are to be held.

Agenda

All meetings should have an agenda, which should be published in good time ahead of the meeting date. Depending on the type of meeting, it may be useful to have a mechanism whereby those attending the meeting can contribute to the agenda items. If that is the case, there should be a deadline in place by which additional agenda items can be submitted.

Minutes and action points

It is traditional to take minutes at meetings and it can be useful to record the minutes of some meetings, but it must be remembered that taking minutes is a skill and my guess is that we have all been in the position of reading minutes that were taken at a meeting we attended that left us wondering if the minutes related to an entirely different meeting. It is always useful to ask the question 'why?': 'Why are we taking minutes?' The answer will probably be, 'Because we need a record of what was said at the meeting'. The second 'why?' is more difficult to answer and if it was responded to would probably elicit a reply something along the lines of 'Because we need records of what the results of the various discussions were'. And yet another 'but why?' may bring the final, exasperated, but all important real reason for taking the minutes and that may well be, 'Because it's important to document what was said in relation to what needs to be done about certain issues, so we need a record of what was agreed and, moreover, we need a record of what was said so it can be referred to at the next meeting'. Those who are tasked with taking minutes at any meeting may like to refer to the following checklist for guidance:

Preparation and planning

- What is the precise purpose of the meeting?
- What overall objective(s) do I have?
- Who will read my minutes?
- How best to record the minutes?
- How can I be sure the information is accurate and reliable?

Writing the minutes

- How should I write and review my minutes?
- What final checks should I make before the minutes are issued?
- Summary

The use of English

- What basic rules in the use of English should I know?
- What common errors in the use of English should I avoid?

Irrespective of whether traditional minutes are taken at a meeting or not, it is far more important to have a set of action points against each topic that was discussed. After each minuted item, following the main discussion points, there should be a note of who is going to do what and by when. With the best will in the world, there will be items that crop up at subsequent meetings that are 'work in hand', but unless there are specific realistic, timed action points, most items on subsequent agendas will remain 'work in hand' and attendees will become disillusioned with meetings.

One of the greatest criticisms one hears about practice meetings is that they are 'talking shops' and no progress is ever made. The chairman's first role is to ensure the discussion centres around the agenda items. A good chairman will ensure that all those attending the meeting have their say on matters that concern them and will be conscious of those who need to be tempered when it comes to contributing to the discussion and of those who need to be encouraged to speak. As far as making progress following meetings goes, having action points that have individuals' names and deadlines against them will go a long way to ensuring this happens. Another common criticism of practice meetings is that they last too long. Ideally, meetings should have both a start and a finish time and it is one of the chairman's jobs to ensure meetings finish on time. It is far better, within reason, to have more frequent, shorter meetings, when minds are fresh and people are keen to contribute, than to have irregular meetings that go on into the night, with everybody doing little else but look at their watches.

REPORTING STRUCTURE

To ensure good communications within a practice, there needs to be a well-defined reporting structure, which is accepted and understood by the team. The reporting structure is there to facilitate the transmission of information in both directions, from the top down as well as from the bottom up. A well-defined, detailed reporting structure, in the form of a schematic or organogram (a chart showing the lines of responsibility between departments of an organization), should go a long way to ensure messages that need to be transmitted are sent through the correct channels to those who need to know. The schematic or organogram should provide details of which topics should be communicated to whom within the practice. For example, where the rota is concerned, everybody in the practice should know whom they need to approach to request a day off or a week's holiday. What tends to happen in too many practices is that those who want to take holidays or a day off at an inconvenient time know only too well the line of least resistance within the practice and approach them with their request, and all too often this can lead to the practice being short staffed, which in turn stresses those who are left working. Far better to have one point of call in the practice, the practice manager, or one of the partners who is the only individual who can sanction time off.

The schematic or organogram should facilitate any member of the team who needs to request or convey a specific piece of information to another individual, a group of people or indeed to the entire team.

ROTAS

The working rota is all too often a source of internal friction and complaints. Time off is precious and those working within the practice team need to know when they are on duty, when they are on call and when they have a long weekend off, etc. Failing to publish the rota well in advance and last-minute changes to the publicized rotas are the biggest sources of friction. It should be feasible at the beginning of each calendar year to complete a master plan for the forthcoming 12 months, indicating who is working which weekend and where possible major blocks of holiday periods as requested by individuals, through having a deadline for submission of requests through the right channels. In some practices there may well be a system in place whereby there is an order in which individuals may select their holidays. For example, in a three-vet practice it may be the year Vet A has the first and sixth choices as to when she takes her holidays, with a maximum of 3 weeks in the summer; Vet B may have the second and fifth choices, leaving Vet C with the third and fourth choices. The following year, everybody moves up the ladder, when this year's Vet C will have the first and sixth choices.

As far as the weekly rota is concerned, it is extremely useful for all concerned, if there can be a rolling 5 or 6 weeks published for all to see. If such a system is in place, it is important for all concerned that requests for all days off, half-days, etc. are submitted to the individual who has the responsibility for drawing up the rotas by a specific date, for example, 2 weeks before the particular day in question. Under this system, to change an already published and circulated rota, except under exceptional circumstances, is fair neither on the individual who draws up the rota nor on the remainder of the team. If an individual does want to alter an already publicized rota, it should be up to that individual to swap with somebody else on the rota, thereby affecting only those two individuals.

INTERPRACTICE COMMUNICATION

There is always the danger of pigeon-holing a book in time, with some contemporaneous comment or other, but I think it fair to say our profession, for the foreseeable future, is going to see an ever-increasing flow of clients travelling between practices. The main drivers behind this traffic are twofold. First, with increasing specialization, the number of clients that are referred is bound to keep growing, and secondly, with the changes in the way out of hours work is now often channelled to practices that are geared up to cope with such work at unsocial hours.

In both cases, the factoring in of another practice, along with clients who may be stressed because of the nature of their animal's condition, makes the need for good communication between practices so important, because there is a greater risk of things not going to plan and the stakes are generally higher if and when they do go wrong.

Interpractice communication can be looked at from two distinct, though related, areas. Firstly, from a business-to-business perspective, and secondly, where the relationship impacts on the clients.

From a business perspective when one practice wants to attract customer from another, whether that be for referrals or for their out-of-hours service, it pays to ensure lines of communication are as efficient as possible. What attracts one practice to 'do business' with another? The main factors are as follows:

- Quality of product or service
- Cost
- Location

When it comes to doing business, especially repeat business, where the quality of competing suppliers is roughly equal, businesses will tend to gravitate to those who make it easy to do business with them; they will take the line of least resistance.

As far as money is concerned, although the cost of a referral or out-of-hours service is nearly always picked up by the client, the first opinion or primary practice may well be involved in explaining the cost of a particular procedure or out-of-hours charge to their own client. Hopefully, the second practice will have played their role in explaining the costs to the clients, making it easier to deal with this situation, should it subsequently arise.

Money can often be a trigger point when it comes to owners complaining, and to mitigate problems in this area, two major things can be done when it comes to interpractice communication. In the first instance, practice B can provide its customer practices with a referral, or out-of-hours pack, which contains both information for the referring practice and information to hand on to clients. As this chapter is devoted to communication between colleagues, suffice it to say that as far as clients are concerned, the information a referring practice will find useful to pass onto its clients is as follows:

- A map with written directions on how to find the referral practice
- A leaflet from the referral practice, describing their business
- An instruction sheet providing details of how and when to present their pet to the referral practice

From the referral practice's perspective, the most important information to get across is about the service it can offer to those who are likely to avail themselves of it. As the American essayist Ralph Waldo Emerson said, 'Build a better mousetrap, and the world will beat a path to your door'. True, but only if they know it exists. So, the first task is to produce a referral pack which can be sent to potential referring practices. Why a pack as opposed to a simple letter and what should this pack contain? It is one thing knowing about the location of the individual who has invented the better mousetrap, but one is not going to beat a path to their door unless you know you have a mouse problem. With that in mind, the pack should contain information aimed at the referring practice team, detailing the services and/or procedures on offer and should include additional information and detail on when it would be advisable to refer. The referral pack should include the wherewithal to make it straightforward, in terms of speed and simplicity, to refer clients. The form can be faxed through to the referral practice or can be given to the client to take with them. My belief is that it will not be long before all this communication will be taking place over the internet.

The referral pack should include a price list that the referring practice can use to provide their clients with estimated costs. As has already been written elsewhere in this chapter, cost can be a major factor when it comes to client satisfaction and niggles, and, where things really go wrong, can be a triggering factor when it comes to complaints and claims. With this in mind, it is vital that the communication of cost and value for money is kept in mind during the entire process of referring clients. This starts with the referring practice and the provision of a rough estimate, a 'ball park' figure. Hopefully, this rough estimate is refined by the referral practice and they keep the client fully informed about the ongoing costs within the referral centre. This whole area of the final cost to the client bearing little resemblance to the initial estimate is all too common, and practices should have the mechanisms in place to keep clients up-to-date with ongoing additional costs.

Having been to the referral or out-of-hours emergency centre, our client will be returning to their home practice for a follow-up consultation. It is vitally important for the clinical history, along with a copy of the client's bill, to arrive at the client's home practice before they do. In the case of the referred client, the practice will hopefully remember they referred their client, but the clients who are seen at the out-of-hours clinic the night before may well turn up at the practice without phoning first. With this in mind, it is most important for the referral or out-of-hours practice to ensure full clinical and financial details of every case seen are communicated to the home practice as soon as possible following the patient's discharge, with the express intention of having those records with the client's own practice before they arrive. Sending details of the case with the client is one method of transferring the information, but this method, on its own, does not provide the necessary forewarning that is so beneficial for all concerned.

A little forethought can save everyone a lot of time and trouble, and can ensure that communication with the returning client gets off to the best possible start. So, in this chapter we have looked at leaders, teams, motivation, meetings and so on, but we have returned to the pivotal aspect of this book, the communication between the veterinary surgeon and the client.

REFERENCES

Donne J (1624) Meditation XVII. In: Donne J, Raspa A (eds), *Devotions upon Emergent Occasions*. Oxford University Press, New York.

Drucker PF (1989) *The Practice of Management*. Butterworth-Heinemann, Oxford.

Maslow AH (1966) *The Psychology of Science: A Reconaissance*. Regnery, Chicago.

Peters TJ, Waterman RH (2004) *In Search of Excellence: Lessons from America's Best-Run Companies*. Harper Business Essentials, USA.

FURTHER READING

Belbin RM (1993) *Team Roles at Work*. Butterworth-Heinemann, Oxford.
Belbin RM (2004) *Management Teams: Why They Succeed or Fail*, 2nd edn. Elsevier Butterworth-Heinemann, Oxford.
Quenck N (1999) *Essentials of Myers-Briggs Type Indicator Assessment*. John Wiley, New York.

Communicating with a wider audience

Jenny Moffett

PUBLIC SPEAKING FOR BEGINNERS

As veterinary professionals, we most commonly communicate with clients and colleagues on a one-to-one basis. However, as with most professions, there will come a time when we will be called upon to talk to larger groups. For vets this may mean holding a herd health evening or presenting a case at a regional clinical meeting. For vet nurses this could include hosting puppy parties, talking to school groups or speaking during practice open days. Even veterinary students, faced with group-learning sessions and clinical rounds, need to learn the basic skills of speaking to groups.

Mark Twain once said, 'There are two types of speakers: those that are nervous and those that are liars'. Nearly 100 years later, public speaking still remains one of people's greatest fears (Figure 7.1). There is, for example, anecdotal evidence to suggest that some individuals are more scared of public speaking than dying (Wallechinsky & Wallace 2005). Why is this? One American survey (Stein et al. 1996), which revealed that one third of people reported excessive anxiety when they spoke to a large audience, reported that the speaker's fears included 'trembling, shaking, or showing other signs of anxiety', 'one's mind going blank', 'doing or saying something embarrassing', 'being unable to continue talking' and 'saying foolish things or not making sense'.

If you tend to avoid public speaking like the plague, it is possible that this could hinder your personal development and career. Whilst an ability to speak in public comfortably widens your career opportunities and makes you more attractive to a potential employer, a proficiency in public speaking has been linked to effective critical thinking as well as academic and professional success (Morreale & Hackman 1994). Grice and Skinner (1995) propose that public speaking is an excellent way of sharpening critical thinking skills such as gathering and recalling, organizing, analysing and evaluating information. In addition, the

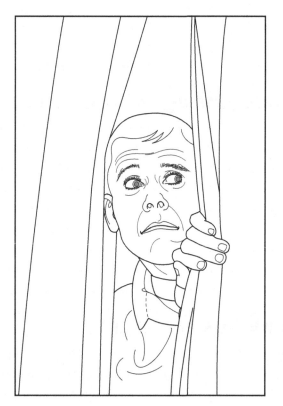

Figure 7.1 Fear of public speaking.

process of 'discovering' your topic, shaping it into a message and delivering it orally are comparable to writing in that it is a learning process (Nicosia 1997).

Preparation: what to say

When it comes to public speaking, Tilton (2002) says, 'Nothing can substitute for quality preparation'. You would not dream of performing your first cruciate ligament repair without reading up on the procedure and making sure that you had all the surgical equipment; an oral presentation needs a similar approach.

Knowing your audience is the first step of this preparation. Before you can plan your presentation, you need to know who will be there to listen to it and why (Petrini 1990; Raveenthiran 2005). You may have organized the presentation or meeting yourself, for example, for a farmer's information night or a practice open day; in this case, you will have some idea of your audience. However, if you have been asked to speak by a third party, such as the local school or a veterinary college, you will need to ask several questions. Ask, who will make up the audience? Do they have any prior knowledge of what I will be talking about and, if so, at what level? What size of a group will be there? It also helps to identify why you have been asked to talk – What do the organizers hope to achieve from the talk? What is the motivation of those attending? Who else will be there and what will they be talking about?

Similarly, you need to decide what message you want to get across – what is the main point of this presentation for you (Petrini 1990)? If it is a practice open day, for example, what do you want to communicate to your audience of clients or potential clients? Do you want to let them know about new facilities, new staff or price changes, or are you simply keen to communicate the quality of the service at your practice? Furthermore, it is useful to identify angles on this message that you are particularly passionate about. A speaker who is enthusiastic about their topic will find it easier to keep their audience's attention.

Once you have identified what message you want to communicate, you can tailor the content of your presentation accordingly. Assessing the right amount and level of information required is important.

Raveenthiran (2005) says it is:

- boring to talk about what the audience already knows;
- futile to talk about what the audience cannot understand;
- arrogant to talk about what you know and ignore the interests of your audience; and
- dangerous to talk about things you are not sure about.

Overfamiliarity of the audience with a topic, says Raveenthiran (2005), gives way to 'contempt'. In other words, do not address a roomful of veterinary radiologists with the basics of how an X-ray machine works. In contrast, unfamiliarity with a topic gives a way to frustration and you risk losing your audience's attention (Raveenthiran 2005; Tilton 2002). Unless you are addressing a group of colleagues, do not use technical terms, jargon or unfamiliar acronyms. If you must use these terms, be careful to spell them out at the beginning of the presentation so that you do not alienate those in the audience who do not understand.

Preparation: how to say it

Rehearsing your presentation is also an important act of preparation (Petrini 1990; Prasad et al. 2000). It may seem time-consuming, but doing a 'dummy run' will help iron out any difficulties and build your confidence. Go through your presentation out loud. This will allow you to proofread your slides for spelling or grammar mistakes, as well as work out whether you are finishing before or after the time limit on your presentation. Try to remember key points, but do not memorize your speech word for word; it is possible that you could go blank (Petrini 1990).

If you perform this rehearsal in front of a mirror, or record it on a video, you will also be able to look at your own body language when delivering the presentation. Watch out for telltale signs of nerves such as crossed legs and arms or wringing hands. Also, if some of your material is particularly complicated or controversial, rehearse it in front of a trusted friend or colleague. Get them to play devil's advocate so that they can highlight what questions or objections to your ideas may arise (Petrini 1990; Prasad et al. 2000). This will reinforce the importance of knowing your topic, especially recent developments or controversial aspects, inside out.

Where practical, performing this dummy run at the actual venue of the presentation is the 'gold standard'. If this is not possible, make sure you know what facilities will be there – Can electronic presentations or slides be used? Are there video and audio facilities? Although it is not helpful to obsess over 'worst case scenarios', having a plan for technical problems, say a computer failure, will help you feel more confident.

Finally, achieving the right frame of mind prior to delivering the presentation is also important. If you are nervous, there are certain techniques such as visualization of a positive outcome, deep breathing and body stretches that can be used to relax (Petrini 1990). Similarly, it can also help to put the presentation into perspective. As oral presentation skills coach James Anderson says, do not let it get out of perspective: 'What's the worst thing that could happen? Even if it does, you'll live. Yes this presentation is important, but it's not brain surgery' (Petrini 1990).

According to communication consultant Gary Cosnett, it is important to set realistic goals for yourself:

> You may set out with the unexamined goal of engaging 100% of the audience 100% of the time. Anyone who's had any speaking experience knows that that's impossible, but many people expect it (Petrini 1990).

Cosnett advises not to 'focus on the 10% or 15% who are not listening' as this takes your attention away from the larger group of people who are listening (Petrini 1990). Also, if you are worried that your nerves will show during the presentation, remember that the audience response is more likely to be empathic rather than hostile or derisive (Petrini 1990).

The presentation as a consultation

Approaching an oral presentation is, in many ways, similar to conducting a consultation with a client. You are there to deliver a message but also to listen to your audience and gauge how they are reacting. Do they look confused? Are they nodding off? Here, it is useful to consider two key factors in the veterinary consultation model (Chapter 2): providing a structure to the proceedings and building a relationship with the client (or audience).

In providing structure to the proceedings, an oral presentation should have a beginning, middle and end that are arranged in a logical sequence (Petrini 1990). An example of this is the concept of: 'Tell them what you're going to say, tell them and then tell them what you have just told them' (Petrini 1990).

A strong opening is important. As Raveenthiran (2005) explains, it is the crucial time to convince your audience that you have something interesting to say. Get your main point out early and give the audience a good reason for being there. A herd health meeting with farmers, for example, may begin with a welcome and a short statement such as: 'Today I'm going to talk about mastitis and the three easiest ways to keep your herd cell count down'. As in a consult, you need to eliminate uncertainty and inform your audience what to expect: 'Today I'm going to talk about BVD. I have a short presentation that should take a half hour and, after a period for questions, we'll break for lunch'.

The end of your speech is also important. If you want your audience to leave with your message resounding in their ears, you need to end on a strong note. Summarize the main points of the presentation or leave the audience with a question. If you end abruptly or dwindle away at the end ('and that concludes my talk on . . .'), your audience may feel somewhat confused or anticlimactic. Some public speaking professionals advocate planning the ending of their presentation first (Petrini 1990). In this way your entire presentation builds up to this final, key message.

Public speaking also reflects the veterinary consultation model in that it is important to build up a relationship with the audience. Creating a rapport will put you, as well as the audience, at ease. The key is to pretend that you are talking to just one person, not a whole audience.

'What makes speakers so nervous is that they haven't connected with the audiences', explains professional speaker Garrison Wynn (Sullivan 2005). So, how do you make this connection? As in a consult, body language is very important; you are not just communicating verbally through your speech and slides, you are also doing so non-verbally, with your body language.

Non-verbal communication with your audience

If you can imagine yourself in conversation with your audience, and adopt body language that appears comfortable and confident, it will help your audience to listen (Natarajan & Kirby 2005). Aim to achieve as open a body posture as possible. This means coming out from behind a lectern, standing up, facing the audience at all times and using open body language – including uncrossed arms and legs. Smile too – audiences appreciate a speaker who appears friendly and enthusiastic.

Eye contact is also key to involving the audience, and not just eye contact with the front row. It may feel rather unnerving at first. Woolf and Kavanagh (2006) suggest:

> Start by finding the person in the audience who is willing you to succeed (there's nearly always one), then look around at the rest of the audience.

Use hand gestures to emphasize interesting or important points and try to move around the stage rather than standing in one place. Do not overdo either, however, and avoid fiddling or fidgeting.

Your voice is another form of non-verbal communication. When you are nervous, your voice naturally speeds up and increases in pitch, so consciously slowing down the rate of your speech will give out a message of confidence and control. Using variation in your pitch and rate of speaking will help prevent you from sounding monotonous. Also, as in a consultation, pauses and short silences can be useful to allow an important piece of information to sink in.

As in a consult, body language is a two-way process. During your presentation, you need to be tuned in to your audience's non-verbal feedback – Do they look bored or confused, for example? Do you need to go over an idea or complicated slide again?

Visual aids

When you give a presentation, visual aids such as charts, tables, graphs, movies and images can help support your speech and keep your audience interested (Petrini 1990). The key to visuals, however, is simplicity. Visuals should support rather than distract from your ideas (Prasad et al. 2000). They should complement your speech rather than replace it – it shows lazy presentation skills to stand in front of an audience and simply read slide after slide verbatim.

Public speaking experts (Essex-Lopresti 1980; Natarajan & Kirby 2005; Petrini 1990; Raveenthiran 2005) have several recommendations for using an electronic presentation application such as Microsoft PowerPoint:

- Use no more than one slide for every 2 minutes of your speech.
- Use contrasting colours, i.e. a light text on a dark blue or black background or vice versa. Care should be taken with red or green because of the potential for red–green colour blindness in the audience.
- Use an appropriate style of text. Universal and Arial are the most popular fonts. Avoid calligraphy, sans serif or italicized fonts. Do not underline text and do not use words or sentences made entirely with upper case letters.
- Use an appropriate size of text. Text should be visible from the back row; try 36 points for titles and 28 points for the body of the text.
- Limit the amount of information on the slide. Sentences should be short and punchy like newspaper headlines. Five points on each slide, consisting of five words each, is a good rule of thumb.
- Ensure there is consistency between slides. Make sure they are the same size, colour, have the same background and that you use the same font throughout.
- Minimize animation and flashy gimmicks such as bullet point sounds. An exception to this is bulleted text. Animating a slide so that a bullet point appears only once the speaker has reached that point is a good way of keeping the audience in time with the speaker.
- Simplify diagrams and use clear, bold pictures. If there are unnecessary elements to a slide, eliminate them.

Any questions?

The question-and-answer session is a valuable part of any presentation. It is the ultimate listening tool for a public speaker that allows you to gain feedback on your performance whilst addressing the needs of the audience. Questions can be taken either during the course of the presentation or at the end. If you are new to the experience, it may be simpler to have the audience save questions for after the talk (Petrini 1990). In this way it will be easier for you to keep on track and on time. Questions should be answered as concisely and clearly as possible, and it is good practice to direct the answer to the entire audience – not just the person that asked the question. When finished, ask: 'Does that answer your question?'

Sometimes you may be faced with tricky questions. Woolf and Kavanagh (2006) say:

People who ask difficult questions often do so to show off their knowledge. These questions often begin, 'Isn't it true that. . .' or, 'But what about . . .' and can often be answered by simply thanking the questioner. Alternatively, ask the questioner for their opinion. They will probably be happy to expound on the subject as this is the reason they spoke up originally.

Similarly, it is important not to react defensively to a question. As Strikwerda (2006) says:

You can 'lose' on information and still win by showing that you're willing to listen, learn, and not lose your cool. The most important thing hostile questioners want is to be heard. If they overdo it and you listen respectfully, you win.

Other useful techniques include asking for the question to be repeated or asking another member of the audience if they would like to answer the question (Woolf & Kavanagh 2006). If all else fails, a simple 'I don't know, but I will find out' is an honest reply.

As you can see, investing a little time in rehearsing for questions, as well as building up a reservoir of facts and logic to back up your arguments (Sullivan 2005), will pay dividends later.

VETERINARY MEDICINE AND THE MEDIA – A MEETING OF TWO WORLDS

Seminars and lectures have their uses, but what if we want to contact an even bigger or wider type of audience? A vet in private practice, for example, may want to highlight a new service to clients or an unusual clinical case to peers. Similarly, a vet involved in research may want to highlight his or her latest findings. Veterinary professionals have the potential to reach enormous numbers of people through the national, regional and local media, as well as to target their message at particular audiences, for example, other vets or researchers.

The media world, in the form of TV broadcasting and print journalism, has not been a traditional habitat for the veterinary profession, but this has changed considerably over the last 10–15 years. An explosion of veterinary programmes such as *Vets' School*, *Vets in Practice*, *Vet Safari* and *Super Vets* has demonstrated a huge public interest in the subject. Although it is easy to write off such media coverage as 'light entertainment', it has several positive features. Aside from helping to open up the profession to the public, the media allows veterinary professionals to promote better animal welfare and responsible pet ownership. It also allows us to give advice and direction on matters of public concern such as food safety and the control of infectious diseases.

On an individual level, working with the media can be used to develop one's career. In academia, for example, the reporting of research findings can enhance citation rates and boost the public profile of research institutions (Phillips et al. 1991). In addition, favourable media reporting can attract political and economic support for research (Salisbury 1997 cited in Allan 2002), whilst in the case of public-funded research, the media can inform the tax-payer how their money is being invested (European Commission 2007a). One only has to look at the amount of money that governments and large corporations invest into advertising and media management to see how importantly they value positive media coverage.

Despite all these opportunities, it has been observed that vets find dealing with the media 'difficult and fraught with danger' (Anon 2007). However, vets are not alone in these perceptions – other scientists and their representative bodies have highlighted an uneasy relationship between their field of expertise and the world of journalism. Research has demonstrated the barriers to reporting science on both sides. A recent EU-wide study (European Commission 2007a), which examined researchers' views of the media, revealed that scientists had a number of negative associations with science reporting. These included the following:

- The belief that the covering of a scientific topic can be driven by imperatives other than the science itself, for example, a political agenda
- The fear that prominence is given to the need to have an attention-grabbing angle at the expense of factual accuracy

- The belief that a modern preoccupation with celebrity culture means that 'popular scientific communicators' are used on scientific topics for which they are not appropriate

The Biotechnology and Biological Science Research Council (Anon 2000) expands on this:

Whereas scientists are concerned with their work and often work to exactitudes and over long periods of times, journalists are working to find the newsworthy angle and to turn a story around in the shortest pace of time. Whilst journalists can see scientists as slow, unhelpful and pedantic, scientists will talk of misrepresentation.

As Gregory and Miller (2000) explain, 'the differences between journalistic and scientific practices can sometimes lead to friction'.

However, science stories can and do make the front page regularly, and once they do, they can have a profound effect on public thinking and individual actions. Entwistle and Hancock-Beaulieu (1992), for example, describe two cases where the media had a direct influence on the health behaviour of individuals. In the first case, press coverage of research which showed links between oral contraceptive use and breast and cervical cancer resulted in a decrease in use of 'the pill'. In the second case, the Bristol Cancer Help Centre experienced a drop in attendees following news coverage of a paper (which proved to be substantially flawed) that suggested that attendance at the centre worsened the prognosis of women with breast cancer.

Press coverage, say Entwistle and Hancock-Beaulieu (1992), also has a huge role in bringing a topic to the table for discussion. 'One unquestioned effect of press coverage', they explain, 'is its powerful role in setting the agenda and stimulating debate about particular issues'. One of the most infamous examples of this agenda setting, in the veterinary field, is the UK bovine spongiform encephalitis (BSE) crisis of the late 1990s.

Case study – how BSE evolved from veterinary to mainstream news

When the first British cow died from BSE, in early 1985, it was an event of veterinary significance only. An unusual neurological condition that bore some resemblance to scrapie, BSE was, initially, 'insufficiently newsworthy' to merit the pages of the national press. For this reason, say Gregory and Miller (2000), media coverage of this new disease throughout the late 1980s, was 'confined to the specialist scientific press and the science pages of the quality daily press'.

The British government's Ministry of Agriculture, Fisheries and Food was first informed about BSE by the Chief Veterinary Officer in June 1987 (Allan 2002). At this stage, little was known about the disease and whether it could be transmitted to humans. However, faced with the prospect of a public health panic and the potential collapse of the livestock export market, the government chose to communicate a message of reassurance: 'British beef is safe'.

Around this time, the government and its veterinary advisors made a number of damaging communication errors. In November 1988, for example, the UK's Chief Veterinary Officer, Keith Meldrum, announced that there was no risk of transmission of BSE to humans through milk. A month later, the sale of milk from cows with BSE was banned. In January 1990, Meldrum proclaimed that BSE was 'not a risk to people'. However, a few days later a research programme to investigate links between cattle and human prion diseases was announced, and Meldrum claimed that it was 'too early' to say that there was no risk to people from BSE (Gregory & Miller 2000). At best, the government and its veterinary department were seen as giving out premature reassurances and, at worst, they were seen as being untruthful. To add to this confusion, several scientific figures were offering opinions that conflicted with that of the government. Professor Richard Lacey, a professor of clinical microbiology at Leeds University, was one of the most vociferous. Professor Lacey, according to Gregory and Miller (2000), said:

> Since the incubation periods for spongiform encephalopathies were in the order of tens of years, no-one would know if people had caught BSE for some time, and that we might find out that an entire generation had been wiped out. The only logical approach for the human population was to avoid all beef products.

The lack of clear-cut, reassuring scientific knowledge, and the conflict of scientific voices, created a degree of uncertainty. This uncertainty can be a valuable tool for the media. As Gregory and Miller (2000) explain:

> In times of uncertainty, it is a clear message that wins the day, both for personal psychological comfort and for social action: it allows us to know both how to feel and what to do.

On 20 March 1996, 'government "spin" was decisively unravelled once and for all' as the then Health Secretary, Stephen Dorrell, announced to members of the House of Commons that there was a 'probable link' between BSE and the human prion disease variant CJD (Creutzfeld–Jakob disease) (Allan 2002). Any trust that the public had in its government and their veterinary advisors was now in tatters.

When it comes to the handling of the BSE crisis, science journalist Jane Gregory Payne (1998) says that there are many valuable lessons to be learnt.

> She explains: 'It is mandatory to provide verified and factual information from a credible source to support emotional and controversial claims during the announcement/definition stage of the media coverage. Without faith in the source of the message . . . or guidance from credible experts, the media tended to seek out explanations which often were based more on speculations than hard science'.

When the scientist's message lacked clarity and credibility, she concludes, 'it invited the press to "fill in the blanks"'.

How to work safely and effectively with the media

As with public speaking, communicating through the media is not unlike communicating with your client in the practice setting – the same verbal and non-verbal skills are important. You should, however, be aware that communicating through the media has introduced a 'middle man' into the equation. Instead of giving your message directly to your client, or target audience, there is now a chain of people between you. Whilst you have a message you need to communicate, it will be done according to the 'rules and constraints' of the world of journalism (Friedman 1986 cited in Allan 2002).

The media, or more correctly the mass media, is a collective term used to describe a method of communication that reaches a large audience. Print media usually refers to newspapers and magazines but also includes directories, newsletters and event programmes. Electronic media includes the internet and broadcast media such as radio or television.

As a veterinary professional, there are two broad reasons for working with the media – either a journalist needs information from you or you have information that you want to communicate to a wide audience, usually via a journalist. Note, however, that there is a growing section of 'media vets' who act as TV figures or writers that bypass this journalist stage (Box 7.1).

Box 7.1 Vet in the public eye

Pete Wedderburn is a small animal practitioner from Bray, Co. Wicklow. He has worked on TV, radio and has several columns in UK and Irish newspapers. Here, Pete shares his experiences of being a vet in the media:

Nine years ago, our receptionist interrupted me between consultations: 'There is someone on the phone from TV3 – can you talk to them?' I did not realize at the time that the subsequent conversation would lead to an entirely new branch in my veterinary career.

Ireland's only independent television channel of the time had recently launched nationwide breakfast time television, known as 'Ireland AM'. The producers of the show had spotted the growing interest in pets in Ireland, and they wanted a vet to come in for a regular 10-minute feature. Would I be interested?

I had already been doing local radio work for a number of years, and the thought of extending this to television appearances was intriguing. After discussing the idea with my partners, I said 'yes', and from that point on, my regular clinic appointments on Wednesdays did not start till 11 AM. Instead, I was busy being on telly.

Television work in Ireland is relatively low key. Viewers are counted in hundreds of thousands rather than in millions, and the performance pressure is similarly toned down. The producers, camera crew and researchers seem very relaxed and unfazed. If there is a small mistake on air, it is not disastrous.

At any level, however, live television is exciting. Sometimes, I find myself looking at the camera and thinking 'What the heck am I going to say now?' Over the years, I have learnt to raise my eyebrows and smile to get over those difficult moments.

Over the 6 years, the format of the show has remained similar. I bring one of my patients into the studio with me. I have 5 minutes to 'show and tell', which gives me a chance to communicate a message about the particular problem of my patient. Once this section is finished, I have 5 minutes to deal with viewer queries. At first, we used to take live phone calls, but it became difficult to prevent the callers from going into lengthy details about their pets' idiosyncrasies. At some point, the producer made the wise decision to take queries in the form of mobile phone texts. These are requested on air half an hour before the vet spot, and I am presented with a list of queries to choose from. The questions are usually simple: 'My Rotty barks 2 much. Wat can I do?', 'Wat shud I feed my Westie puppy?', but occasionally, they can be more challenging: 'My dog has Alopecia X. What treatment do you recommend?'

There is no rehearsing, and it is always 'ad libbed'. There is the continual possibility of absolute disaster in front of hundreds of thousands of people, yet somehow, that is part of the fun. I know that it is not living on the edge in the same way as climbing mountains or paddling down the Amazon, but in its own way, it does give me a weekly internal injection of adrenaline.

The weekly preparation for the show is simple. Every Tuesday, I get a phone call from the television researcher. What am I bringing in the following day? I have spent the week scanning my patients for television suitability. The television team generally leave this choice up to me, and over the years I have covered most aspects of pet care and common diseases. Fat cats, balding dogs, dentistry, skin tumours, cataracts: these subjects may seem mundane to vets, but to the public, every case is new and interesting. As I explain the case over the phone to the researcher, they type up notes for the presenters, and when I arrive the next day, the television team has been briefed and everything is ready for me to walk onto the set.

I have an early start every Wednesday, leaving home at 7.00 AM and collecting my patient-of-the-week on the way to the television studios. I take the pets in my own car, usually without the owners. Most folks have to go to work, and they are delighted to lend me their animals for their 15 minutes of fame. I always need to reach the studios well in advance of my appearance time. I am not renowned for good time-keeping, but when live television is involved, there is no room for lateness. I usually arrive an hour before I am due to go on. This allows plenty of time for preparation and for unexpected incidents such as traffic delays.

While I am waiting for my slot each week, I am called into the make-up room. My pale, tired, pasty face is manipulated by an efficient, friendly lady with brushes and powders. Within minutes, I have every appearance of having just returned from a 2-week holiday in the sun. It is a pleasant session of gentle pampering. Even my eyebrows are carefully combed and my hair is subtly gelled and positioned. It is the only time in my life that my appearance receives such close attention. Once the show is over, I am supposed to remove the make-up with baby wipes, but it is easy to forget, and I am sure some of my clients must give me odd looks on these occasions. Why is the vet wearing make-up?

The weekly television appearance does mean that I am well known in a very vague way by the public in Ireland. Most folk who recognize me cannot remember where they have seen me before. Much as I would love them to swoon and say 'Oh, the TV vet!', the most common comments are 'Where have we met before?' or 'How do I know you?' There are times when it is not so good to be easily recognized. I was once asked to open a pet shop in a town in the middle of Ireland. As I left at the end of a busy day of pet talk, I told my wife how relieved I was to be leaving 'Pete the Vet' behind so that I could relax. When we arrived at the hotel, and a fellow guest said loudly, 'Aren't you the vet from the television?', I was forced to present the 'Pete the Vet' persona again, which was exactly what I did not feel like doing. I will never need sunglasses and a hat to hide from legions of fans, but there are just a few occasions when anonymity would be a blessing.

The most enjoyable aspect of television work is the variety of new challenges that it injects into my weekly work routine. I have to come up with an interesting new angle to present to the viewers every week. I need to negotiate with pet owners to arrange for their pets to feature beside me. And, on the day, I have to arrange my thought processes clearly so that I can send out the message that I want to pass on, rather than the mumbled vagueness which could easily come out of my mouth when under pressure. I also enjoy working with a range of colleagues in the media who live in an entirely different world to my normal veterinary sphere. They have their own jargon, with terms such as OB (outside broadcast), LVO (live voice over) and PTC (piece to camera). And yes, people really do say 'It's a wrap'. There is definitely a perceived glamour in television work, and although the rate of pay is generally no better than much veterinary work, it can be fun mingling with 'media types' and bumping into occasional genuine 'celebrities'.

When looking for a science or veterinary story, journalists get their information from several sources, which include journals, meetings, press conferences and press releases, as well as from more general breaking news stories, unsolicited calls and their own sources (Greenberg 1997 cited in Allan 2002).

If you have information you need to communicate via the media then you will need to make the initial approach. The usual way to do this is by releasing the information in a traditional format, such as a media or press release, or by contacting a journalist directly. However, as with public speaking, preparation of how you choose to communicate your information is essential.

If you have information that you want to be used as a news story, you should ask yourself the two following questions:

1.   What do you hope to achieve?
2.   How do you hope to achieve it?

If we take the example of a veterinary practitioner who is launching a new canine hydrotherapy pool at his practice, we can look at what sort of answers these questions might receive.

What do you hope to achieve?

- We would like to make more people – clients and other veterinary practices – aware of the new facilities.
- We would like to attract more clients to use the facilities.
- We would like to encourage our existing clients to use the facilities.
- We would like to make more people aware of the benefits of canine hydrotherapy.

How do you hope to achieve it?

- We will place an advertisement in a local paper.
- We will get editorial coverage in the local newspaper.
- We will get coverage on the local radio channel.
- We will send a brochure out with all of this year's vaccination reminders.

These two basic questions form the bones of a communication plan, which you can use to locate which medium you want to target. If, as in the above-mentioned example, you have a local interest story, your ideal targets would be the local newspapers and radio stations – perhaps even a regional TV station. If you want neighbouring practices to know that they can refer a dog to your hydrotherapy clinic, the national veterinary press may also be appropriate. If you are working in the field of veterinary research, your story may find a home either in the specialist scientific press or in the wider, national press – depending on its newsworthiness (see below).

Remember, competition for news coverage can be high, and you have to convince journalists that you have a story worth telling, with the minimum of effort on their part. So how do you do this?

What makes a good story?

There are two main ways of framing a story in the media – either as a hard news article or as a feature article (Randall 2007). A hard news article is generally short, fact-based and to-the-point. Usually, the most important points of the story (e.g. what happened, when, where and to whom?) are covered in the first few sentences. Feature stories, on the other hand, are generally longer and have more freedom of expression. However, for a piece of information to merit translation into either a hard news article or a feature article, it must be what we call 'newsworthy' or have 'news values' (Randall 2007).

But what is newsworthiness? As the old adage, accredited to US journalist and author Charles A. Dana, says: 'If a dog bites a man, that's not news. But if a man bites a dog, that's news!'

When it comes to science stories, as many veterinary stories are framed, there are several journalistic criteria that make up newsworthiness. A recent EU-wide (European Commission 2007b) study highlighted the following as the most important:

1. Relevance – the news item must be relevant to everyday life.
2. Novelty – a news item must tell something not previously known.
3. Understandable – a news item must be easy to understand and mean something to the reader.
4. Proximity – news which relates to the particular country where a newspaper or TV station is based is more newsworthy.
5. Political or controversial – many journalists look for a political angle to a story.
6. Sensation and originality – stories that can 'touch' readers are more newsworthy.

Other news values (Rensberger 1997 cited in Allan 2002) include reliability of the results, i.e. whether the scientific work is from a reputable source, and timeliness. Time is of the essence in news circles and news should as up-to-date as possible. The turnaround on news articles can be extremely quick, and journalists often work to deadlines that are in the order of hours or even minutes.

The newsworthiness of a story is often increased if one can find a human angle (Allan 2002). Taking the example of our vet with the hydrotherapy pool, a journalist would view the option of an interview with a satisfied client, or a veterinary nurse that works at that clinic, as an attractive addition to the story.

Similarly, a good quality image can also make the difference between an article being published and rejected (Anon 1999; Martineau 2007). Most publications require high-resolution digital images that are well lit and not blurred. Further to this, pictures of people and animals are much more welcome than those of items or buildings (Anon 1999).

Forming a media release for veterinarians

Once you have an idea of the story you want to tell, you must now reproduce it in a format that is easily recognizable to a journalist. Typically, this means drawing up a media (or press) release – a piece of written communication, which is emailed or faxed to journalists and editors at newspapers, magazines and/or TV or radio broadcasting networks.

A media release (Figure 7.2) should include the following parts (Anon 2000; Martineau 2007; PRWeb 2007):

- Announcement – 'press release' or 'media release' usually appears at the top of the document. *(1)*
- Headline – this is used to grab the attention of the reader and briefly summarize what the release is about. *(2)*
- Subheading – a single sentence under the headline, which expands on the content of the release. *(3)*
- Date – when the release has been sent. *(4)*
- Location – where the release has come from. *(5)*
- Introduction – this explains briefly the major points of the news release, for example, Who? Where? What? Why? *(6)*
- Body – this represents the second and subsequent paragraphs of the release, which contain greater detail about the piece of news, i.e. further explanation, statistics, background or other relevant details. As with other forms of communication to a non-technical audience, try to avoid jargon, acronyms and long words. *(7)*
- Contact information – this includes a designated media contact who is willing, able and available to take media enquiries. Details should include the job or title of the person (so as to put them into context), along with his or her phone number, fax number and email and postal addresses. If there is a relevant website, include this too. *(8)*
- Notes to editor – this includes brief background information on the people, events or organizations mentioned in the story. If you have photos, add 'photos available on request' at this point. If you are emailing your release, you can attach one good example to catch the journalist's interest. *(9)*
- End – to indicate that the media release has come to an end, it is normal convention to write the symbol '###' and/or the word 'ends'. *(10)*

A media release is designed to catch, and hold, the reader's attention. In the same way that a CV should be tailored to a potential employer, a media release should be tailored to its specific media target. With our canine hydrotherapy example, a media release to the local newspaper, for example, could concentrate on the people and location of the clinic, whilst a release tailored to a national veterinary magazine may concentrate more on the facilities available and the actual hydrotherapy. Also, as with a CV, the information should be kept short and to-the-point, and the important points should not be 'hidden' at the bottom of the release. If a release is to be used and needs to be shortened, newspaper and magazine editors tend to cut from the bottom upwards (Anon 2007).

Finally, as discussed above, finding a human angle is important. In a media release, a quote from one or two sources will help to give the piece 'colour'. Keep the quotations short as, according to Chambers (2006), 'quotes which are short and concise are more likely to be printed, and printed in their entirety'.

MEDIA RELEASE *(1)*

Water therapy first for poorly pooches *(2)*
New Enniskillen hydrotherapy facility represents a first for dogs in Northern Ireland.
(3)

July 10, 2008. For immediate use *(4)*
Enniskillen, Co. Fermanagh, Northern Ireland *(5)*

A vet has launched the first hydrotherapy facility for dogs in Northern Ireland. The
Canine Rehabilitation Clinic, set up by Richard Hamilton, practice principal at Forest
Veterinary Practice, Enniskillen, was opened on July 10, 2008. *(6)*

The clinic, situated adjacent to the existing Forest Veterinary Practice premises, is
open to dogs of all ages and breeds. Appointments can either be made through the
practice or following referral from other veterinary practices.

Hydrotherapy, a popular form of medical treatment in humans, is a growing therapy
for animal species. During a hydrotherapy session, the dog is placed in a pool
of warm water. The temperature of the water allows muscles to relax, easing pain and
stiffness, making it easier for the dog to exercise. The water also supports the dogs,
which gives their joints support and protection while they exercise. Hydrotherapy is
especially useful in relieving painful joints and increasing the range of movement in
joints and improving muscle strength.

Speaking at the launch of the clinic, Mr Hamilton said: 'I am delighted that we now
have such a facility up and running in Enniskillen. It is an incredibly valuable tool to
help in the rehabilitation of animals after surgery or after car accidents so it's a real
boon to the practice.' *(7)*

For further information contact:
Richard Hamilton
Forest Veterinary Practice
13 Ballyroan Street
Enniskillen
Co. Fermanagh
BT74 3LW

Tel: 0044 28 6565 3334
Fax: 0044 28 6565 3333
Email: rhamilton@forestvets.co.uk
Web: www.forestvets.co.uk *(8)*

Notes to editor:

Forest Veterinary Practice is a six-vet practice that was established in 1999. Vets at
the practice specialize in companion animal medicine and see clients with cats, dogs,
rabbits and other pets. Practice principal Richard Hamilton qualified from the Royal
Veterinary College, London in 1981. He has a specialist qualification in veterinary
surgery.
Attached photos shows practice principal Richard Hamilton with three-year-old
Labrador Spike and Spike's owner, Laura Moore. A range of photos taken at the
launch are available on request. *(9)*

ENDS ### *(10)*

Figure 7.2 An example of a media release for a local newspaper.

Now that you have created your media release, you need to use it as effectively as possible. First, you must locate the best destination for it. If you are drawing up a news story for your local paper, call the news office to find out how they prefer to receive stories, for example, by email or fax. Then find out the contact details of the news editor and send it directly to them. You can also post your press release on a commercial press release distribution service such as 'AlphaGalileo' (www.alphagalileo.org) or on your practice or personal website, if you have one (Martineau 2007). After you have sent out your media release, make follow-up telephone calls to ensure that it has reached its destination. Be prepared to resend it as releases can often get lost or mislaid.

Second, you must choose the most appropriate time to release the story. If possible, avoid busy news periods, for example, around a governmental budget or general election. This will increase your chances of getting published or broadcast. You can also use an embargo to your advantage. An embargo is a date and/or time issued along with a press release, which informs the media when a story can go to press. Mark this clearly at the top of the press release: 'embargoed until ...'. The Biotechnology and Biological Sciences Research Council (BBRSC) (Anon 2000) recommends using an embargo to increase your chances of publication:

> Towards the end of the week journalists are often looking for stories for Monday editions of programmes and papers. Providing them beforehand with something embargoed for Monday may increase the chances of your release being used.

If you do not want to place an embargo on your release, mark it as available 'for immediate use' (Figure 7.2 (4)). Whether you place an embargo or not, do make sure that the contact you mention on the release is available immediately (Anon 2007) and has not, '[disappeared] for a two-week conference in the middle of nowhere' (Anon 1999).

Media interview skills

A successful CV often leads to an interview, and so too does a successful press release. If your release is sufficiently newsworthy, you may be contacted by a journalist, seeking further information via an interview.

Interviews can take many forms – they can be carried out in person or over the phone, and they can be used to write an article or produce a TV or radio piece (either prerecorded or live). They can also be short and to-the-point or longer and more in-depth.

Whether your interview is being recorded for television or over the phone, it is akin to public speaking: preparation is essential (Anon 2000; Royal Society 2000). You need to give some consideration to what you want to say and how you want to say it. When someone calls to set up an interview, find out some basic information about the set-up of the interview – what will be the line of questioning or, even better, what questions will be asked? Will the interview be live or recorded? Who else, if anyone, is appearing? How long will the interview take? What level of audience will this be aimed at – what publication does the journalist represent? If the interview is to be broadcast, will it be as part of a scientific programme or a 'human interest' programme?

As with giving a presentation, you should decide in advance on your key messages – what do you want to get across? If your topic is somewhat controversial, it is also wise to prepare for tricky questions. Imagine being interviewed by a competitor or someone who disagrees with your opinion – what sort of questions would they want to ask you?

In addition, consider how the public will perceive you. Even if you are being interviewed on a non-veterinary matter, your job or practice will mean that you are seen as a representative of the veterinary profession. Because of this there are certain recommendations, such as those of your professional body, to take into consideration. The Royal College of Veterinary Surgeons (RCVS) (2006), for example, says:

> [V]eterinary surgeons must ensure that any statement is factually correct, distinguishing clearly between personal opinion or political belief and established facts ... They should be careful not to express or imply that any view is shared by the profession at large unless previously authorised by the RCVS, BVA or other professional body.

If you are to be interviewed on television, another part of preparation is your physical appearance. Think about how you want to come across: neat, professional attire is usually best (Science Media Centre 2007). Achieving the right body language is also important. As with public speaking, it is usually best to adopt an open, relaxed appearance. Sitting or standing with uncrossed arms and legs, whilst achieving good, consistent eye contact with the interviewer, are the basic guidelines. Try not to worry about the camera and concentrate on speaking with as normal a tone, pace and pitch as possible.

When it comes to the content of the interview, make sure that you are making sense to the interviewer. Do not speak in technical jargon, even to an industry specialist (Anon 2007), and if you must use big words, explain them. Also, be aware of what you want to have reported and what you do not. There can be some confusion about journalistic conventions such as being 'on' or 'off' the record. As the Department for Business, Enterprise and Regulatory Reform (formerly known as the Department of Trade and Industry) explains (Anon 1999):

> Even journalists can get confused about what is 'off the record' (what you say is not to be used, so it is best not to say anything on this basis) and 'unattributable' (use it but don't say who told you).

If you are in any doubt about mentioning something, do not (Royal Society 2000).

In some situations, vets as scientists may be called on to discuss a controversial or 'breaking news' story, which can bring extra challenges. If you are cold called by a journalist in the light of an emerging news story, it is good practice to ask for 10 minutes to retrieve something to refer to, and collect your thoughts (Anon 1999). Remember, however, that the journalist may be working to a tight deadline and you may need to keep the delay brief. Ask the journalist about their deadline and their subject, and then call them back or give them a time to call you back (Anon 1999).

The most difficult types of interviews are those which involve controversial subjects or uncertain areas of science. The Science Media Centre (2006), an independent organization that helps scientists to work with the news media, has several guidelines when it comes to controversy:

- Do not be afraid to say 'We simply don't know'.
- Stay calm. Be honest, frank and open.
- Do not be afraid of saying that something is not 100% safe.

- Avoid ducking the question.
- Think about what your audience needs to know – address their concerns.

The Royal Society (2000) advises interviewees not to feel pushed into an answer:

Although a reporter may want a straightforward yes or no answer, don't be pressurized into making a response that you will later regret. If you do not know the answer to a particular question, say so. Never lie.

Ensuring that you have prepared yourself thoroughly and taking the few simple guidelines above into consideration can make the media interview as stress free a procedure as possible.

REFERENCES

Allan S (2002) *Media, Risk and Science*. Open University Press, Philadelphia, PA.

Anon (1999) *Going Public: An Introduction to Communicating Science, Engineering and Technology*. DTI Publications, London.

Anon (2000) *Communicating with the Public*. Biotechnology and Biological Sciences Research Council, London.

Anon (2007) Dealing with the media spotlight. *Veterinary Record* 160(15):495.

Chambers D (2006) 'Killer virus arrives': how Defra press releases regarding avian influenza were processed by the written press and interpreted by the public. MSc thesis, Liverpool University, UK.

Entwistle V, Hancock-Beaulieu M (1992) Health and medical coverage in the UK national press. *Public Understanding of Science* 1:367–382.

Essex-Lopresti M (1980) Illuminating an address: a guide for speakers at medical meetings. *Medical Education* 14:8–11.

European Commission (2007a) European research in the media: the researchers' point of view. Report, European Commission. December 2007.

European Commission (2007b) European research in the media: what do the media professionals think? Report, European Commission. December 2007.

Gregory J, Miller S (2000) *Science in Public: Communication, Culture and Credibility*. Perseus, New York, pp. 176, 243.

Gregory Payne J (1998) Media coverage of the mad cow issue: introduction. In: Ratzan SC (ed.), *The Mad Cow Crisis: Health and the Public Good*. New York University Press, New York, p. 134.

Grice GL, Skinner JF (1995) *Mastering Public Speaking*. Allyn and Bacon, Boston.

Martineau N (2007) How do I write a press release? SciDevNet. Available online: http://www.scidev.net/en/practical-guides/how-do-i-write-a-press-release-.html (accessed 5 September 2008).

Morreale SP, Hackman MZ (1994) A communication competency approach to public speaking instruction. *Journal of Instructional Psychology* 21(3):250.

Natarajan A, Kirby JA (2005) A guide to oral presentation skills. *Student British Medical Journal* 13:353–396. Available online: www.studentbmj.com/issues/05/10/careers/376.php (accessed 5 September 2008).

Nicosia G (1997) Implementing public speaking skills across the curriculum. *Community Review* 15:74–81.

Petrini CM (1990) A survival guide to public speaking. *Training and Development Journal* 44:15–25.

Phillips DP, Kanter EJ, Bednarczyk BT, Tastad, PL (1991) Importance of the lay press in transmission of medical knowledge to the scientific community. *New England Journal of Medicine* 325:1180–1183.

Prasad S, Roy B, Smith M (2000) The art and science of presentation: electronic presentations. *Journal of Postgraduate Medicine* 46:193–198.

PRWeb (2007) Tips, guidelines and templates for writing an effective press release. Available online: www.prwebdirect.com/pressreleasetips.php (accessed 5 September 2008).

Randall D (2007) *The Universal Journalist*, 3rd edn. Pluto Press, London.

Raveenthiran V (2005) The 10 commandments of oral presentations. *Student British Medical Journal* 13:353–396. Available online: www.studentbmj.com/issues/05/10/careers/374.php (accessed 5 September 2008).

RCVS (2006) *Guide to Professional Conduct*. RCVS, London.

Royal Society (2000) Scientists and the media. *Guidelines for Scientists Working with the Media and Comments on a Press Code of Practice*. Royal Society, London.

Science Media Centre (2006) Communicating risk in a soundbite: a guide for scientists. Available online: http://www.sciencemediacentre.org/uploadDir/admincommunicating_risk.pdf (accessed 18 September 2008).

Science Media Centre (2007) Top tips for media work: a guide for scientists. Available online: http://www.sciencemediacentre.org/pages/publications/ (accessed 18 September 2008).

Stein MB, Walker JR, Frode DT (1996) Public speaking fears in a community sample: prevalence, impact on functioning, and diagnostic classification. *Archives of General Psychiatry* 53:169–174.

Strikwerda C (2006) Jokes and quote: tips on public speaking for hardworking deans. *Academic Leader* 22(2):5–6.

Sullivan VK (2005) Public speaking: the secret weapon in career development. *USA Today* May:24–25.

Tilton JE (2002) Adventures in public speaking: a guide for the beginning instructor or public speaker. *FBI Law Enforcement Bulletin* February:15–19.

Wallechinsky D, Wallace A (2005) *The Book of Lists*. Canongate Books Ltd, Edinburgh.

Woolf K, Kavanagh J (2006) Giving presentations without palpitations. *British Medical Journal Career Focus* 332:242–243.

Communication and self-care in the veterinary profession

Communication, stress and the individual

Martina A. Kinsella

Things which matter most must never be at the mercy of things which matter least.

(Goethe)

The veterinary profession fails to talk aloud about the 'internal struggles' and 'demons' it experiences (Connolly 2004). Therefore, what we have today among veterinarians is a profession with an unacceptable level of suicide, mental illness, alcoholism and drug addiction (Mellanby 2005). With respect to suicide, recent research by Bartram et al. (2009) has highlighted a range of factors which may predispose members of this profession to such behaviour, including high levels of anxiety and depressive symptoms, higher 12-month prevalence of suicidal thoughts, less favourable psychosocial work characteristics, lower levels of positive mental well-being and higher levels of negative work–home interaction.

A prerequisite for admission into a veterinary degree course is to be a gifted and highly intelligent student. Maintaining such an elevated existence right through veterinary training, alongside the competitive nature of vet school, inevitably sows the seeds of extreme expectations that vets will continue to demand from themselves in their working career. This, attached to the seemingly endless list of professional demands and sources of stress (Table 8.1), can have far-reaching consequences for those not equipped with the necessary skills to cope (Halliwell & Hoskin 2005; Voracek 2004).

Further to the role of being a veterinarian, there is life off the job to contend with. Technological advances such as laptops and mobile phones mean one is never far from the job. Role conflict may arise as a result when:

the attitudes, values and behaviours required for one role, may be incompatible with those needed in another. These opposing behavioural expectations may create tension within individuals as they make the transition from one environment to another.

(Cooper et al. 2001)

Table 8.1   Multiple sources of stress and professional demands in the veterinary profession

Workload	Client Issues	Workplace Interpersonal Relationships
Overwork	Difficult or demanding clients	Staff relations
Excessive task demands	Unreasonable clients' attitudes	Problems with peers
Being on call	Complaints	Lack of support
After-hours work	Unhappy clients	Staff management (for managers)
Time pressure	Clients' poorly controlled animals	Difficulties with management for employees
Deadlines	Unreliable/unpunctual clients	Organizational communication
Long hours/days	Concerns over clients' finances	Mistakes
	Dealing with clients' grief	
	Criticism	

Work Outcomes	Work Constraints	Other Stressors
Unsuccessful treatments	Paperwork	Own feelings of inexperience
Difficult cases	Poor equipment or facilities	Desire to do the best job possible
	Bureaucracy	Desire to keep skills up-to-date
	Involvement with other agencies	Financial concerns
	Audits	Balancing work and family commitments
	Unclear accountabilities	High level of responsibility
	Work interruptions	Risk of litigation
	Social isolation	Travel
	Monotony	Physical demands
	Repetitive work	Weather
	Lack of career advancement	Organizational changes

Reproduced with kind permission from Gardner (2005).

THE FIRST STEP TO INNER FREEDOM

What lies behind us and what lies before us are tiny matters, compared to what lies within us.

(Oliver Wendell Holmes)

Recognizing and embracing the complexity of being human, one's own individuality, combined with both inherited and acquired personality traits is an invaluable starting point in discovering the pathway to inner freedom. Although there are many external factors contributing to the problems for veterinary professionals, the state of the inner mind, its deep-rooted thinking and natural responses have the capacity to determine whether a situation is either a good or bad experience for the vet. Additionally, the tendency to suffer stress and its severity can be measured by careful analysis of the emotional, physical and behavioural symptoms of stress. Table 8.2 serves as a good indicator in determining the intensity of one's own stress levels.

Table 8.2 Recognizing the symptoms of stress

Emotional Symptoms	Physical Symptoms	Behavioural Symptoms
Anxious/nervousness	Dry mouth	Impatience
Anger/frustration	Restlessness/uptight	Hyperactivity
Mood swings	Palpitations	Aggressiveness
Irritability	Nausea/vomiting	Accident-prone
Tearfulness	Muscle tension/cramps	Smoking more
Loss of humour/enjoyment	Pain/increased illness	Substance/alcohol abuse
Isolation	Fatigue/loss of energy	Poor performance/work
Lack of confidence	Weakness/dizziness	Absenteeism
	Butterflies in stomach	Uncooperation
	Diarrhoea/constipation	Compulsive–obsessive behaviour
	Loss/increase of appetite	Loss of sex drive

Source: Kinsella (2006).

MOVING FROM VICTIM TO VICTOR

Internal dialogue has the ability to be either constructive or destructive to the human spirit. Messages of doom and gloom, critical self-analysis, fear, anxiety, thoughts of failure, feelings of inadequacy, low self-esteem/value, and so on, will undoubtedly create a state of consciousness that is crippling to achieving. The obvious result is exactly this – non-achievement. Thus, the reinforced negativity sends another spiral of negative messages to the brain, further compounding the previous. A self-fulfilling prophecy develops, where negative thoughts give rise to negative feelings, resulting in negative outcomes. The person is convinced that they were right all along – they knew it would go wrong and it did. This sets the pattern for future problems if not corrected (McGraw 2004; Needleman 1999).

Roet (2000) stated that if we give minimal attention to the possibilities of a situation, and live our life by the probabilities, there is a greater chance the possibilities we feared might never happen. For example, the vet is called to a sick animal urgently. The probability is he/she will call out, examine, diagnose, attend and treat the animal for the illness it suffers and all will be well. The possibilities could be that the vet gets a puncture on the way and, in the panic, breaks the expensive bottle of medication required for the animal. They are delayed for an hour and the animal deteriorates (or has died) by the time they arrive. The vet might make an improper diagnosis, and if the farmer is aware of this, they could conclude that this vet is incompetent, convincing the vet of the fears and low self-value they already believe about themselves. The chances are that a negative approach to any given situation will serve as a very strong influence in obtaining the wrong outcome. Of course, one must not be naïve in thinking that things will not ever go wrong, and that thinking positively about situations will automatically see them right. No, what is being said is to be aware at a level, one must be prepared for the unexpected occurring and that personal effort is required in most situations. However, balanced thinking and not giving too much weight to problems prior to them happening, but dealing with them as they arise, is a far better approach and less draining on the mind and body. According to Needleman (1999), there are a number of factors likely to contribute to self-defeating behaviours and response patterns being maintained by individuals:

1. Individuals may be unaware of adaptive strategies relating to their problems. Failure to find adaptive strategies can arise from high levels of physiological arousal, and extreme levels hinder thinking, creativity and effective problem solving.
2. Self-fulfilling prophecies. Negative expectations influence people's responses; their responses in turn result in their expectations being fulfilled.
3. Ongoing negative treatment by others, particularly significant others, can eventually lead to individuals forming negative core beliefs that perpetuate their distress.
4. Anxiety resulting from a belief that they would become an entirely different person by giving up a long-term pervasive strategy. Fear causes people to strongly resist attempting new approaches to their difficulties.
5. Individuals with ongoing problems may feel hopeless with regard to their ability to change self-defeating patterns. Previous attempts to change may have been unsuccessful in the past, thus feelings of hopelessness can mean lack of motivation in attempting change.
6. Maintaining self-defeating patterns as a result of immediate reinforcing strategies. Consequences that follow immediately after a behaviour tend to have a more powerful effect on subsequent behaviour than do consequences that are delayed. For example, the immediate, although short-term, relief from depression that some can derive from alcohol can be sufficient to keep the individual drinking to excess – despite the fact that it may make the depression worse over the long term.
7. Maladaptive behaviour patterns are often reinforced intermittently. An intermittently reinforced maladaptive pattern is much harder to stop if occasionally it is seen by others/society as good. For example, passive people sometimes gain positive praise about their 'nice quiet personality' from colleagues, to keep them from speaking out against behaviour they do not agree with.
8. Social environments can unintentionally reinforce maladaptive behaviour patterns. For example, a person receiving more support and attention when depressed could continue the maladaptive behaviour for the continuation of support and attention.
9. Some self-defeating behaviours and response patterns are encouraged and reinforced by society at large. Work-alcoholism can come from society's preference for success and the hunger for material possessions serves to drive people to live beyond their means. Alcohol and drugs can be seen as 'cool' in society, thus individuals may constantly use these to 'fit in'.

IMPLEMENTING CHANGE

It does not matter how the wind blows, the only thing that matters is how you set your sail.

(Peiffer 1999)

The human mind is the most fascinating and mysterious creation conceivable. It has the capability to withstand numerous difficulties and sometimes horrendous experiences against all the odds, yet its capacity to self-destruct or suffer a complete battering in seemingly smaller, less upsetting situations serves to remind us that effective self-management plays a primary role in the growth and evolution of the mind. According to Covey (1999), there are four dimensions of renewal necessary for us to effectively manage ourselves. These include the following:

1. Physical – which involves eating proper food, rest, relaxation and regular exercise.
2. Spiritual – comprising commitment to your values. This is your core, it is very private, drawing upon your sources of inspiration that uplift and join you to beliefs about humanity.
3. Mental – entailing our learning through formal education, interesting programmes, books, etc.
4. Social/emotional – this implicates others in our lives, interpersonal relationships, cooperation and communication along with showing consideration for other people around us.

Our ability to communicate effectively can only develop through self-awareness – being transparent with the deeply embedded and engrained value systems that we have developed over time. So how might this be done? 'Thought is one of the greatest faculties that God gave to us human beings' (Peale 1998). Therefore, understanding oneself lies in deliberately observing, exploring and employing energy into our patterns of thinking. Particular attention to our automatic thoughts is paid, then to the feelings that emerge from our thinking and finally to the behaviour that results from our feelings. This need not be a very big exercise, but through habitually practising the exploration of self, positively rewarding discoveries manifest themselves. Many people, however, are unclear what is meant by feelings. Table 8.3 displays a number of examples of feeling words to help the reader identify his/her own experience.

By simply keeping a daily record over a period, it is possible to investigate contributing factors to our personality traits. These valuable techniques can be an asset to people in transforming their attitudes. If followed by a commitment to learning new ways of being and integrating them in life, many more rewarding skills will ensue, such as tremendous self-confidence, assertiveness skills and the ability to speak with conviction, thus transforming one's life. Figure 8.1 is a thought evaluation worksheet, followed by a sample form (Figure 8.2), a thought evaluation worksheet that shows some sample ideas for keeping records (Needleman 1999).

Table 8.3 Feeling words

Types of Feelings	Feelings Words
Happy feelings	Calm, confident, content, curious, ecstatic, focused, interested, loved, playful, proud, relaxed
Feelings of sadness	Alone, anxious, bored, detached, disappointed, discouraged, exhausted, helpless, indifferent, lonely, miserable, numb
Feelings of anger	Aggravated, aggressive, angry, annoyed, disgusted, frustrated, furious, hurt, impatient, jealous, mean, mischievous, resentful, torn
Feelings of fear	Crazy, envious, paranoid, resistant, scared, shocked, shy, sceptical, surprised, terrified, worried

Adapted from Tindall (1994).

Triggering stimuli	Thinking	Feelings	Behaviour

Figure 8.1 Thought evaluation worksheet.

Applying your own experience to the sample sheet, attempt to record in the four columns how the situation lies with you, in other words, what triggers your thinking, the feelings that follow and how these feelings impact on your behaviour. You may record negative experiences only or negative and positive experiences on the same or separate sheets. Recording both negative and positive opens your awareness to corrective methods of dealing with negativity. According to Burns (1999), 'Sometimes the vulnerabilities we try so hard to hide can be our greatest asset in terms of getting close to others'. Being closer to others gives greater scope for requesting help when in difficulty.

LEARNING ASSERTIVENESS SKILLS AND BECOMING AN ASSERTIVE INDIVIDUAL

Half the misery in the world comes of want of courage to speak and to hear the truth plainly, and in the spirit of love.

(Harriet Beecher Stowe)

According to Tindall (1994):

Assertiveness skill enables one to stand up effectively for one's own dignity, respect and courtesy without violating the rights of others while at the same time helping others to recognise and more completely obtain their rights.

Triggering stimuli	Thinking	Feelings	Behaviour
Department inspection due	He will see I'm no good, I always mess up, I'm useless.	Anxious Worried	Become nervous, forget important things. Perform poorly.
Ring girlfriend and she's too busy to talk right now	Why doesn't she want to talk with me? My mother never had time to talk with me either.	Anger Sceptical	Retract intimacy, behave in a cold manner, withdraw and be angry with all women.
Some colleagues head out together for lunch	They don't want me or they would have asked me along. I'm too boring, a loser.	Upset Hurt Disappointed	Be uncooperative and refuse to help them. Stay moody and annoyed all day, beating yourself up about the situation.
Assigned extra work in practice with horses	I know a lot about horses, I grew up with them, I love horses and can do very well with them.	Delighted Focused Interested Proud	Confident work, enjoy performing tasks and company of owners, perform exceptionally well.
Boss asks you to come see him	He's going to criticize me. He may stop me doing some calls or cut my wages.	Fear Resentment Anger Paranoid	Talk fast, not really listening or concentrating on anything. Maybe pick up the wrong message. Or Go quiet, say nothing, tremble inside holding an outer front of bravery.
Sun is shining	I love the sun, it makes me feel good, I enjoy the heat.	Happy	Perform tasks much easier, great work done and feel really good.
Last call/task of the day	Great I'm off tonight, I can go home meet my family and friends and have a good time.	Calm Relaxed Excited feeling inside	Stress disappears, much more relaxed. Job doesn't seem quite so bad after all.

Figure 8.2 Sample thought evaluation worksheet.

Once an individual has established a clearer picture of their thoughts, feelings and behaviour patterns whether by using the above-suggested thought evaluation worksheet or by another method more suited to their needs, they will then be more equipped for behaving assertively and reflecting when dealing with other people. An assertive person will be more specific about their wants and needs, having carefully decided whether their requests are impinging upon the rights of other people. Honesty, openness, self-esteem and clarity all develop further, with each successful experience at practising assertiveness. Appropriate criticism can be accepted more readily and seen by the listener as a learning curve rather than a put-down. Aggressive or passive behaviour can very often be the response from non-assertive individuals, leaving a trail of hostility and bad feeling behind it.

Many factors influence a person's likelihood of attaining an assertive personality. Family background and the people we grow up with are predominantly responsible for teaching us productive life skills. Love, understanding and appraising the positives, while respectfully pointing out areas that may be letting us down, build a solid foundation in influencing our emotional growth (Lindenfield 2001). However, all is not lost if we did not have the ideal start in life. It is possible to train ourselves and satisfactorily learn assertiveness. There are some widely recognized and helpful pointers used by educators and trainers in preparation for assisting people in assertiveness training courses. These include speaking calmly, expressing your feelings and beliefs directly and honestly, 'owning' them by using 'I' statements, maintaining good eye contact and standing up for your rights in a respectful manner (Tindall 1994).

Here are some examples of assertive expressions in comparison to aggressive and passive expressing.

I feel upset when you say I am no help to you because I have made a huge effort, even working overtime to clear the backlog. Your lack of appreciation completely undermines me as a person. (Assertive)

You ungrateful so and so, can't you see how much work I have done, even working over time to clear the backlog? Maybe if you did a little more yourself instead of sipping cups of tea we wouldn't ever have a backlog? (Aggressive)

I am really sorry because I thought my overtime was useful in clearing the backlog. I'll try harder from now on, would that be helpful? (Passive)

Modelling assertive behaviour, constantly rehearsing and practising this new way of being is a liberating experience. The most rewarding thing is, together with the advantages for oneself, many other people will see you as a role model for them, so make sure you are a good one.

Creating and cultivating a culture of self-care, self-analysis, acknowledgement of self as OK, and learning self-assertiveness, will eventually lead to good communication, thus helping to release the snares that so tightly bind the voice of vets, keeping them silent about their inner turmoil and distress. It is up to veterinary professionals to 'plant the seed and the universe will give you the tree. Be careful what seeds you sow!' (Reynolds 2000).

Beyond words: communication, social relationship and health

David Bartram

There is no agony like bearing an untold story inside you

(Hurston 2006)

If Only They Could Talk, James Herriot's first volume of veterinary adventures (Herriot 1970), implies his regret of the diagnostic limitations imposed by animals' inability to speak, but it could equally lament the emotional inarticulacy of some veterinary professionals and the consequences for their mental and physical health.

On the basis of proportional mortality ratios in England and Wales (Kelly & Bunting 1998; Mellanby 2005) and Scotland (Stark et al. 2006), and similar estimates in the USA (Miller & Beaumont 1995), Australia (Jones-Fairnie et al. 2008) and Norway (Hem et al. 2005), veterinary surgeons appear to be at particularly high risk – around four times more likely than the general population to die by suicide and approximately twice as likely than other health care professionals.

While many factors are likely to influence the suicide rate in the veterinary profession (for a review, see Bartram & Baldwin 2008), work-related stress is likely to play an important role. Veterinary work is perceived as stressful by over 80% of UK veterinary surgeons (Robinson & Hooker 2006). Using a short, validated stress evaluation tool to measure and compare a number of work-related stressors and stress outcomes across occupations in the UK, Johnson et al. (2005) showed that veterinary surgeons reported lower psychological well-being than most other occupations. A cross-sectional survey of work-related stress in the veterinary profession in New Zealand (Gardner & Hini 2006) showed that of those working in small animal and mixed practice, women and younger veterinarians reported the highest levels of stress, primarily associated with long working hours, clients' expectations and unexpected clinical outcomes. Other possible sources of stress include after-hours on-call duties, relationships with peers, managers and clients, lack of resources, emotional exhaustion or 'compassion fatigue' (due to, for example, euthanasia of animals and dealing with clients' grief), inadequate professional support, travelling for ambulatory duties, concerns about maintaining skills, personal finances, making professional mistakes and the possibility of clients' complaints and litigation.

Communication can have adverse and beneficial effects on health. Communication in the context of interpersonal conflicts or in giving bad news to animal owners, in relation to euthanasia of companion animals (Ptacek et al. 2004), compulsory slaughter of livestock or advising of a poor medical prognosis for example, can be stressful events for veterinary surgeons. In contrast, disclosing information, thoughts and feelings about traumatic, stressful or emotional events (self-disclosure), has been found to result in improvements in both psychological and physical health, in non-clinical and clinical populations. This chapter reviews some of the empirical research into those beneficial effects and offers a number of strategies for enhancing our health and happiness through more effective communication.

THE DISCLOSURE PHENOMENON

When people transform their thoughts and feeling about personally upsetting experiences into language, consistent and significant physical and mental health improvements follow. Individuals who were victims of violence and who kept this experience silent were significantly more likely to have adverse health effects than those who openly talked with others (Pennebaker & Susman 1988). In short, having any type of traumatic experience is associated with elevated illness rates; having any trauma and not talking about it further elevates the risk.

If keeping an upsetting experience secret is unhealthy, can talking about it, or in some way putting it into words, be beneficial?

Most studies which compare writing alone to talking either into a tape recorder (Esterling et al. 1994) or to a therapist in a one-way interaction (Donnelly & Murray 1991; Murray et al. 1989) find comparable biological, mood and cognitive effects. Talking and writing about emotional experiences are both superior to writing about superficial topics. Speaking has the added benefit of allowing an additional mode of emotional expression – vocal expression – that may arouse more emotions and increase task involvement more than verbal expression alone (Murray & Segal 1994), but on the basis of existing research, writing and talking probably have similar outcomes for people's health and well-being (Lyubomirsky et al. 2006). By contrast, merely thinking about traumatic life events does not result in beneficial outcomes. The search for meaning and understanding that typically follows the experience of a traumatic event, although deemed necessary and beneficial, has the potential to degenerate into rumination, a series of negative, repetitive and intrusive thoughts. Numerous studies have documented that self-focused rumination produces a host of adverse outcomes (Lyubomirsky & Tkach 2004).

Interestingly, a systematic analysis of positive events can be counterproductive as it removes any uncertainty or mystery around positive experiences, transforming them from something surprising, thrilling and extraordinary into something mundane, ordinary and less emotionally intense; thinking repetitively about positive events can, however, be beneficial for the individual (Lyubomirsky et al. 2006).

Pennebaker and Chung (2006) suggest the following instructions for using expressive writing as a therapeutic tool:

For the next 4 consecutive days, write for a minimum of 15 minutes continuously a day on your deepest thoughts and feelings about an extremely important emotional issue that has affected you and your life.

In your writing, really let go and explore your very deepest emotions and thoughts.

You might tie your topic to relationships with others, to your past, your present or your futures, who you would like to be or who you are now.

You may write about the same general issues or experiences on all days of writing or about different topics each day.

Do not worry about spelling, grammar or sentence structure. You can write by hand or you can type on a computer. If you are unable to write, you can also talk into a tape recorder.

All of your writing is completely confidential and no feedback will be given.

The immediate impact of expressive writing is usually a short-term increase in distress, negative mood and physical symptoms, and a decrease in positive mood compared with controls. However, at long-term follow-up, many studies have continued to find evidence of health benefits in terms of objectively assessed outcomes and self-reported physical and emotional health outcomes. For example, Baikie and Wilhelm (2005) found the following longer-term benefits of expressive writing:

- Health outcomes
  - Fewer stress-related visits to the doctor
  - Improved immune system functioning
  - Reduced blood pressure
  - Improved lung function
  - Improved liver function
  - Fewer days in hospital
  - Improved mood/affect
  - Feeling of greater psychological well-being
  - Reduced depressive symptoms before examinations
  - Fewer post-traumatic intrusion and avoidance symptoms
- Social and behavioural outcomes
  - Reduced absenteeism from work
  - Quicker re-employment after job loss
  - Improved working memory
  - Improved sporting performance
  - Higher students' grade point average
  - Altered social and linguistic behaviour

Expressive writing may be most effective at least 1–2 months after an upheaval, and the benefits occur even if the writing is not read by anyone else (Pennebaker and Chung (2006).

Proven benefits of expressive writing

A meta-analysis of 13 studies using expressive writing by healthy participants (Smyth 1998) suggests that for physically and psychologically healthy individuals, the effects produced are similar in magnitude to the effects of other psychological interventions, many of which are more involved, time-consuming and expensive. In clinical populations, a meta-analysis of 9 studies (Frisina et al. 2004) found a significant benefit for health. The effect was stronger for physical than for psychological health outcomes. A recent meta-analysis of 146 studies (Frattarolli 2006) supports these observations.

How does expressive writing work?

Although the exact mechanism by which expressive writing confers health benefits is still unclear, there have been a number of potential explanations. There is probably not a single mediator.

There is little support for the initial hypothesis that expressive writing operates through a process of emotional catharsis or venting of negative feelings. Although experiencing emotions while writing is a necessary component of the expressive writing effects, writing only about the emotions associated with a trauma is not as beneficial as writing about both the event and the emotions (Pennebaker & Beall 1986).

Another possible explanatory theory is inhibition (Pennebaker & Beall 1986). Actively inhibiting thoughts and feelings about traumatic events requires effort, serves as a cumulative stressor on the body and is associated with increased physiological activity, obsessive thinking or rumination about the event and longer-term disease. Confronting a trauma through talking or writing about it, and acknowledging the associated emotions, is thought to reduce the physiological work of inhibition, gradually lowering the overall stress on the body. Such confrontation involves translating the event into words and enabling understanding, which further contributes to the reduction in physiological activity associated with inhibition and rumination. This theory has intuitive appeal but mixed empirical support. Although inhibition may play a part, it does not completely explain the benefits.

Pennebaker and Chung (2006) advance an analogue-to-digital conversion theory to explain the emotional processing effects of disclosure: verbally labelling an emotion is much like applying digital technology (language) to an analogue signal (emotion and the emotional experience). It is hypothesized that if an emotion or experience remains in analogue form, it cannot be understood or conceptually tied to the meaning of an event. The only way by which an emotion or experience in non-linguistic form can leave awareness is through habituation, extinction or the introduction of a new or competing emotion. Once an experience is translated into language, it can be processed in a conceptual manner in which an individual can assign meaning, coherence and structure. This allows for the event to be assimilated and ultimately resolved and/or forgotten, thereby alleviating the maladaptive effects of incomplete emotional processing on health.

This analogue-to-digital theory of processing emotions through language is supported by observations using computerized text analysis systems (Pennebaker et al. 2001) to explore the use of positive and negative emotion words (happy, sad), causal words (because, reason) and insight words (understand, realize) in relation to various health outcomes. The development of a coherent narrative over time, reflecting increasing cognitive processing of the experience, helps to reorganize and structure memories of traumatic experiences and appears to be critical in enabling an individual to reach an understanding of a problem and in changing their perspective. Written language demands more integration and structure than spoken language.

Disclosure leads to further disclosure – writing encourages people to talk openly with others about their experiences.

IMPORTANCE OF SOCIAL RELATIONSHIPS

The centrality of social connection to our health and well-being cannot be overstated. Humans are powerfully motivated by a pervasive drive to seek out and maintain strong, stable and positive interpersonal relationships (Baumeister & Leary 1995). Most scientists would agree that a desire to form and preserve social bonds has an evolutionary basis. Human beings would not have been able to survive or reproduce without such a motivation.

There is considerable evidence that social factors such as social support and social integration are associated with health outcomes (Cohen 2004). Social support refers to a social network's provision of psychological and material resources intended to benefit an individual's ability to cope with stress. Social integration (or connectedness) refers to participation in a broad range of relationships.

Social support is often differentiated into three subtypes: instrumental, informational and emotional. Instrumental support involves the provision of material aid, for example, financial assistance or help with daily tasks. Informational support refers to the provision of relevant information intended to help the individual cope with current difficulties and typically takes the form of advice or guidance in dealing with one's problems. Emotional support involves the expression of empathy, caring, reassurance and trust and provides opportunities for emotional expression and venting. All forms of social support are important, and veterinarians have been shown to make good use of their social networks to seek out information and assistance in solving work-related problems, especially from 'informal' networks such as family, friends and work colleagues more than resources such as mentors, professional associations and helplines (Gardner & Hini 2006).

There are a number of reasons why veterinary professionals might feel isolated, such as relocation, unsupportive work colleagues or employers, shyness or simply the constraints of a demanding on-call rota. New graduates in particular can feel the shock of relocating to an area where they do not have ready personal and professional support networks. They have previously been surrounded by fellow students during their undergraduate course and may suddenly find themselves in an unfamiliar small town or rural location with few friends or colleagues near for company (Stobbs 2004). We all need to be able to share our thoughts, feelings, successes and failures with someone who cares. Stobbs (2004) recommends the strategies listed in Box 8.1 for coping with isolation. The mechanisms through which social relationships influence health are summarized in Table 8.4.

Box 8.1   Strategies for coping with isolation

- Try to realign your thinking towards the positive present and future outcomes of your relocation.
- Get to know colleagues better by showing an interest in their families and hobbies.
- Try to negotiate the on-call rota so that you can have the same evening off each week to pursue a hobby or join a class where you can make new friends.
- Make lots of acquaintances rather than just one close friend. If you forge a close relationship with somebody, make sure you do not neglect your relationships with others.
- Establish and maintain professional links by attending study days, conferences and meetings, especially if you are working in a small practice.
- Maintain your links with family and old friends by phone and email.
- Book time off in advance for holidays and meetings with friends and family.
- If there is discord or lack of support in the workplace, discuss the issues with your colleagues or employers, maintain your own sense of self-worth and keep your links with other professional colleagues to help buffer you against any feeling of alienation.

Reproduced with permission from Stobbs (2004).

Positive effects on health

Striking evidence for stress buffering in the physical health realm is reported in a prospective study of healthy Swedish men aged 50 years and over (Rosengren et al. 1993). Those with high numbers of stressful life events in the year before the baseline examination were at substantially greater risk for mortality over a 7-year follow-up period. However, this effect was ameliorated among those who perceived that high levels of emotional support were available to them. In contrast, perceived emotional support made no difference for those with few stressful events.

Table 8.4 Mechanisms through which different types of social constructs influence physical health

Social Construct	Mechanism	Specific Processes
Social support	Stress buffering	Eliminates or reduces effects of stressful experiences by promoting less threatening interpretations of adverse events and effective coping strategies.
Social integration	Main effect (independent of stress)	Promotes positive psychological states (e.g. identity, purpose, self-worth and positive effect) that induce health-promoting physiological responses. Provides information and is a source of motivation and social pressure to care for oneself.
Negative interactions	Relationships as a source of stress	Elicits psychological stress and in turn behaviour and physiological concomitants that increase risk for disease.

From Cohen (2004).

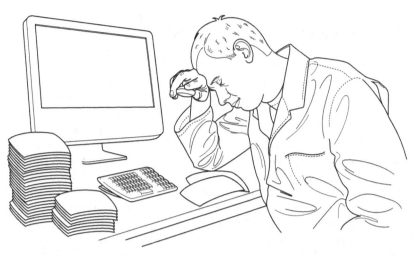

Figure 8.3 Despair.

Social connectedness is beneficial irrespective of whether one is under stress or not. DeLongis et al. (1988) showed that people with unsupportive social relationships were more likely to experience an increase in psychological and physical health problems both on and following stressful days, even if they generally have little stress in their lives. The benefits come through the promotion of positive psychological states and the effect of social controls and peer pressures that influence normative health behaviours. For example, social networks might influence whether an individual takes exercise, has a healthy diet, smokes or takes illicit drugs. Role concepts that are shared among a social network help to guide interaction by providing a common set of expectations about how individuals should act in different roles. In meeting these normative role expectations, individuals gain a sense of identity, predictability and stability, of purpose, and of meaning, belonging, security and self-worth. These positive thoughts and emotions are presumed to be beneficial because they reduce psychological despair (Figure 8.3), result in greater motivation to care for oneself, or result in suppressed neuroendocrine response and enhanced immune function (Cohen 2004).

An association between social integration and reduced mortality has been replicated in many studies (reviewed by Berkman & Glass 2000), and other studies have found that greater integration predicts survival from heart attacks, less risk for cancer recurrence, less depression and anxiety and less severe cognitive decline with aging (Cohen et al. 2000). Furthermore, social integration has been shown to confer resistance to infectious illness. Cohen et al. (1997, 2003) showed that active participation in social roles reduces susceptibility to developing a cold after experimental challenge with common cold viruses. Although sociability is associated with more and higher-quality social interactions, it predicted disease susceptibility independently of these variables and independently of immunity to the viruses at baseline. A recent, large pan-European study (Knesebeck & Geyer 2007) confirmed that emotional support is positively associated with self-rated health.

Developing and maintaining close personal relationships affects psychological well-being more than any other single factor. Diener and Seligman (2002) in their study of the upper 10% of consistently very happy people found a key difference between the happiest and less happy groups. The very happy people had rich and satisfying social relationships with friends, family and a romantic partner, spent the least time alone and the most time socializing. The authors conjectured that good social relationships are universally important to human mood. It is not known whether rich social lives cause happiness or if happiness causes rich social lives, but it is interesting that social relationships form a necessary but not sufficient condition for high happiness – that is, they do not guarantee high happiness, but it does not appear to occur without them.

Negative effects on health

Social environments and one's responses to them can have powerful detrimental effects. Social isolation can be a stressor in its own right, increasing negative effect and a sense of alienation, loneliness and stress while decreasing feelings of control and self-esteem. There is also growing evidence for neuroendocrine changes and alterations in immune response induced by a lack of social support (Berkman & Glass 2000).

Further, social conflicts can also increase susceptibility to disease. Subjects with enduring problems with spouses, close family members and friends were more than twice as likely to develop the common cold after experimental challenge as persons without any chronic stressors in their lives (Cohen et al. 1998).

THE ROLE OF TELEPHONE SUPPORT HELPLINES

Sometimes, rather than sharing our distressing thoughts with those known to us, we may prefer to speak to someone anonymously and in complete confidence, what TS Eliot described (in his play, *The Cocktail Party* 1949) as 'the luxury of an intimate disclosure to a stranger'.

The effectiveness and utility of telephone helplines are generally well established. One measure of the effectiveness of such services has been the assessment of suicide rates in communities served by the centres. In England, Bagley (1968) compared suicide rates in 15 towns with suicide centres with the rates in two samples of towns which were matched for sociodemographic variables and did not have such centres. He also compared the rates during 3 years before and 3 years after the establishment of the centres. He found that there was a decline in suicide rates in the towns with suicide prevention centres compared to control towns, which experienced an increase in suicide rate. Lester (1997) conducted a meta-analysis of studies that presented data as to whether suicide prevention centres prevented suicides in the communities served. Twelve of the 13 studies reported a preventive effect, although the effect failed to reach statistical significance in one, and in many the size of the effect was small. When the results for each of the studies were combined, a significant preventive effect was identified.

Helplines (Figure 8.4 and Table 8.5) vary in the type of support provided. Support generally takes the form of active listening (e.g. validation of emotions, reframing, moral support, reflection of feelings and showing understanding) and/or collaborative problem solving

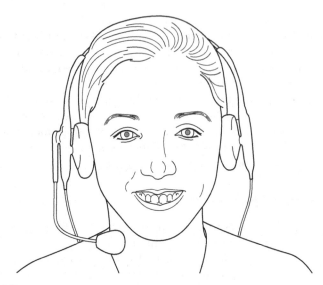

Figure 8.4 Helplines.

(e.g. asking fact questions on the problem, questioning about resources and discussing possible ways to solve the problem) (Mishara et al. 2007).

A less directive approach involving active listening was significantly related to reduction in suicidal urgency for new callers; with repeated callers there may be greater benefits from using a more directive approach (Mishara & Daigle 1997), such as collaborative problem solving.

Kalafat et al. (2007) demonstrated significant decreases in non-suicidal callers' crisis states and hopelessness during the course of the telephone session, with continuing decreases in the following weeks. In the same study, Gould et al. (2007) demonstrated significant decreases in the suicidality of suicidal callers, with continuing decreases in hopelessness and psychological pain in the following weeks.

Table 8.5 Examples of available telephone helplines

Telephone	Contact
Vet Helpline	07659 811 118 (UK)
A 24-hour peer-support telephone helpline service staffed by trained volunteers	
Samaritans	08457 909 090 (UK)
'Listening' emotional support for people with feelings of distress or despair, including those which could lead to suicide	
Befrienders Worldwide	Contact telephone numbers for many countries can be obtained from the website www.befrienders.org
Works worldwide to provide emotional support and reduce suicide	

SUMMARY AND CONCLUSIONS

The purpose of this chapter has been to provide an overview of the empirical evidence for the mental and physical health benefits associated with communication and social connectedness.

Not talking about a traumatic experience is associated with a breakdown of one's social network, a decrease in working memory, sleep disruptions, substance misuse and an increased risk for further traumatic experiences. Expressive writing or the unfettered talking about trauma can often short circuit this process (Pennebaker & Chung 2006).

Talking or writing forces people to stop and re-evaluate their life circumstance and enables thoughts and images to be integrated into a coherent narrative. Language is, by its nature, highly structured. Speaking or writing prompts us to think in causal terms (e.g. A may have led to B, which may have led to C), thereby triggering an analysis that can help us find meaning, enhanced understanding and, ultimately, a sense of control. When an experience has structure and meaning, it seems much more manageable and controllable than when it is represented by a chaotic and painful jumble of thoughts and images. Translating emotional experiences into words demands a different representation of the events in the brain, in memory, and in the ways people think on a daily basis. As recent studies have indicated, this can bring benefits including improved mood and enhanced immune function.

All these cognitive changes have the potential for people to come to a different understanding of their circumstances. The cognitive changes themselves now allow the individuals to begin to use their social worlds differently. They talk more; they connect with others differently. They are now better able to take advantage of social support. And with these cognitive and social changes, many of their unhealthy behaviours abate (Pennebaker & Chung 2006).

There is much truth in the old adage that 'a problem shared is a problem halved'. Translating emotional experiences into words, whether by means of expressive writing, talking to those in our social networks or sharing our thoughts and feelings with a stranger via a telephone helpline, is not a panacea but it is an effective and readily available coping tool.

ACKNOWLEDGEMENTS

David Bartram gratefully acknowledges the contribution of Professor James W. Pennebaker of the psychology department of the University of Texas at Austin for his comments on the draft manuscript.

REFERENCES (COMMUNICATION, STRESS AND THE INDIVIDUAL)

Bartram DJ, Yadegarfar G, Baldwin DS (2009) A cross-sectional study of mental health and well-being and their associations in the UK veterinary profession. *Social Psychiatry and Psychiatric Epidemiology* March 18. details [Epub ahead of print].
Burns David D (1999) *The Feeling Good Handbook*. Penguin Books, Harmondsworth, UK.

Connolly D (2004) Stress in the veterinary profession. *Irish Veterinary Journal* 57: 315–316.

Cooper CL, Dewe PJ, O'Driscoll MP (2001) *Organisational Stress – A Review and Critique of Theory Research and Applications.* Sage Publications, London.

Covey SR (1999) *The 7 Habits of Highly Effective People.* Simon & Schuster, UK Ltd, London.

Gardner D (2005) *Work Demands, Coping, Satisfaction and Stress Among Veterinarians.* School of Psychology, Massey University, New Zealand.

Halliwell REW, Hoskin BD (2005) Reducing the suicide rate among veterinary surgeons: how the profession can help. *Veterinary Record* 157(14):397.

Kinsella M (2006) *Self-Care and Stress Management.* Lecture, University College Dublin, Ireland.

Lindenfield G (2001) *Assert Yourself.* Thorsons Publishers, Hammersmith, England.

McGraw P (2004) *Family First.* Simon & Schuster, UK Ltd, London.

Mellanby RJ (2005) Incidence of suicide in the veterinary profession in England and Wales. *Veterinary Record* 155: 415–417.

Needleman LD (1999) *Cognitive Case Conceptualization.* Lawrence Erlbaum Associates, New Jersey.

Peale NV (1998) *The Positive Way to Change Your Life.* Vermilion, Ebury Press, Random House, London.

Peiffer V (1999) *Positive Thinking.* Element Books, New York.

Reynolds Q (2000) *Intuition – Your Secret Power.* Adventures in Astonishment Publishers, Dublin.

Roet B (2000) *The Confidence to Be Yourself.* Judy Piatkus Publishers, London.

Tindall JA (1994) *Peer Power: Becoming an Effective Peer Helper and Conflict Mediator.* Accelerated Development Publishers, Indiana.

Voracek M (2004) National intelligence and suicide rate: an ecological study of 85 countries. *Personality and Individual Differences* 37 (3): 543–553.

FURTHER READING (COMMUNICATION, STRESS AND THE INDIVIDUAL)

Humphreys T (1996) *The Family – Love It and Leave It.* Gill & Macmillan, Dublin.

Humphreys T (2000) *Work and Worth – Take Back Your Life.* Gill & Macmillan, Dublin.

Humphreys T (2002) *Examining Our Times – for the Way We Live Now.* Gill & Macmillan, Dublin.

REFERENCES (BEYOND WORDS: COMMUNICATION, SOCIAL RELATIONSHIPS AND HEALTH)

Bagley G (1968) The evaluation of a suicide prevention scheme by an ecological model. *Social Science and Medicine* 2:1–14.

Baikie KA, Wilhelm K (2005) Emotional and physical health benefits for expressive writing. *Advances in Psychiatric Treatment* 11:338–346.

Bartram DJ, Baldwin DS (2008) Veterinary surgeons and suicide: influences, opportunities and research directions. *Veterinary Record* 162:36–40.

Baumeister RF, Leary MR (1995) The need to belong: desire for interpersonal attachments as a fundamental human motivation. *Psychological Bulletin* 117:497–529.

Berkman LF, Glass T (2000) Social integration, social networks, social support, and health. In: Berkman LF, Kawachi I (eds), *Social Epidemiology*. Oxford University Press, New York, pp. 137–173.

Cohen S (2004) Social relationships and health. *American Psychologist* 59:676–684.

Cohen S, Doyle WJ, Skoner DP, Rabin BS, Gwaltney JM, Jr (1997) Social ties and susceptibility to the common cold. *JAMA* 277:1940–1944.

Cohen S, Doyle WJ, Turner R, Alper CM, Skoner DP (2003) Sociability and susceptibility to the common cold. *Psychological Science* 14:389–395.

Cohen S, Frank E, Doyle WJ, Skoner DP, Rabin BS, Gwaltney JM, Jr (1998) Types of stressors that increase susceptibility to the common cold in adults. *Health Psychology* 17:214–223.

Cohen S, Gottlieb B, Underwood L (2000) Social relationships and health. In: Cohen S, Underwood L, Gottlieb B (eds), *Measuring and Intervening in Social Support*. Oxford University Press, New York, pp. 3–25.

DeLongis A, Lazarus RS, Folkman S (1988) The impact of daily stress on health and mood: psychological and social resources as mediators. *Journal of Personality and Social Psychology* 54:486–495.

Diener E, Seligman MEP (2002) Very happy people. *Psychological Science* 13:81–84.

Donnelly DA, Murray EJ (1991) Cognitive and emotional changes in written essays and therapy interviews. *Journal of Social and Clinical Psychology* 10:334–350.

Eliot TS (1949) The cocktail party. In: Eliot TS (ed). (2004) *The Complete Poems and Plays*. Faber, London.

Esterling BA, Antoni MH, Fletcher MA, Margulies S, Schneiderman N (1994) Emotional disclosure through writing or speaking modulates latent Epstein–Barr virus antibody titers. *Journal of Consulting and Clinical Psychology* 62:130–140.

Frattarolli J (2006) Experimental disclosure and its moderators: a meta-analysis. *Psychological Bulletin* 132:823–865.

Frisina PG, Borod JC, Lepore SJ (2004) A meta-analysis of the effects of written emotional disclosure on the health outcomes of clinical populations. *Journal of Nervous and Mental Disease* 192:629–634.

Gardner DH, Hini D (2006) Work-related stress in the veterinary profession in New Zealand. *New Zealand Veterinary Journal* 54:119–124.

Gould MS, Kalafat J, Munfakh JLH, Kleinman M (2007) An evaluation of crisis hotline outcomes Part 2: suicidal callers. *Suicide and Life-Threatening Behavior* 37:338–352.

Hem E, Haldorsen T, Aasland OG, Tyssen R, Vaglum P, Ekeberg O (2005) Suicide rates according to education with a particular focus on physicians in Norway 1960–2000. *Psychological Medicine* 35:873–880.

Herriot J (1970) *If Only They Could Talk*. Michael Joseph, London.

Hurston ZN (2006) *Dust Tracks on a Road: An Autobiography*. Harper Perennial Modern Classics, New York, p. 176.

Johnson S, Cooper C, Cartwright S, Donald I, Taylor P, Millet C (2005) The experience of work-related stress across occupations. *Journal of Managerial Psychology* 20:178–187.

Jones-Fairnie H, Ferroni P, Silburn S, Lawrence D (2008) Suicide in Australian veterinarians. *Australian Veterinary Journal* 86(4):114–116.

Kalafat J, Gould MS, Munfakh JLH, Kleinman M (2007) An evaluation of crisis hotline outcomes Part 1: nonsuicidal crisis callers. *Suicide and Life-Threatening Behavior* 37:322–337.

Kelly S, Bunting J (1998) Trends in suicide in England and Wales, 1982–96. *Population Trends* 92:29–41.

Knesebeck O, Geyer S (2007) Emotional support, education and self-rated health in 22 European countries. *BMC Public Health* 7:272.

Lester D (1997) Effectiveness of suicide prevention centres – a review. *Suicide and Life-Threatening Behaviour* 27:304–310.

Lyubomirsky S, Sousa L, Dickerhoof R (2006) The costs and benefits of writing, talking and thinking about life's triumphs and defeats. *Journal of Personality and Social Psychology* 90: 692–708.

Lyubomirsky S, Tkach C (2004) The consequences of dysphoric rumination. In: Papageorgiou C, Wells A (eds), *Rumination: Nature, Theory, and Treatment of Negative Thinking in Depression*. Wiley, Chichester, UK, pp. 21–41.

Mellanby RJ (2005) Incidence of suicide in the veterinary profession in England and Wales. *Veterinary Record* 155:415–417.

Miller JM, Beaumont JJ (1995) Suicide, cancer and other causes of death among California veterinarians, 1960–1992. *American Journal of Industrial Medicine* 27:37–49.

Mishara BL, Chagnon F, Daigle M, Balan B, Raymond S, Marcoux I, Bardon C, Campbell JK, Berman, A (2007) Comparing models of helper behavior to actual practice in telephone crisis intervention: a silent monitoring study of calls to the US 1–800-SUICIDE network. *Suicide and Life-Threatening Behavior* 37:291–307.

Mishara BL, Daigle M (1997) Effects of different telephone intervention styles with suicidal callers at two suicide prevention centers: an empirical investigation. *American Journal of Community Psychology* 25:861–895.

Murray EJ, Lamnin AD, Carver CS (1989) Emotional expression in written essays and psychotherapy. *Journal of Social and Clinical Psychology* 8:414–429.

Murray EJ, Segal DL (1994) Emotional processing in vocal and written expression of feelings about traumatic experiences. *Journal of Traumatic Stress* 7:391–405.

Pennebaker JW, Beall S (1986) Confronting a traumatic event: toward an understanding of inhibition and disease. *Journal of Abnormal Psychology* 95:274–281.

Pennebaker JW, Chung CK (2006) Expressive writing, emotional upheavals, and health. In: Friedman HS, Silver RC (eds), *Foundations of Health Psychology*. Oxford University Press, New York, pp. 263–284.

Pennebaker JW, Francis ME, Booth RJ (2001) *Linguistic Inquiry and Word Count (LIWC)*. Erlbaum Publishers, New Jersey.

Pennebaker JW, Susman JR (1988) Disclosure of traumas and psychosomatic processes. *Social Science and Medicine* 26:327–332.

Ptacek JT, Leonard K, McKee TL (2004) I've got some bad news …: veterinarians' recollections of communicating bad news to clients. *Journal of Applied Social Psychology* 34:366–390.

Robinson D, Hooker H (2006) *The UK Veterinary Profession in 2006: The Findings of a Survey of the Profession Conducted by the Royal College of Veterinary Surgeons*. RCVS, London.

Rosengren A, Orth-Gomer K, Wedel H, Wilhelmsen L (1993) Stressful life events, social support and mortality in men born in 1933. *British Medical Journal* 307:1102–1105.

Smyth JM (1998) Written emotional expression: effect sizes, outcome types, and moderating variables. *Journal of Consulting and Clinical Psychology* 66:174–184.

Stark C, Belbin A, Hopkins P, Gibbs D, Hay A, Gunnell D (2006) Male suicide and occupation in Scotland. *Health Statistics Quarterly* 29:26–29.

Stobbs C (2004) Isolation in the workplace: taking control, finding a way forward. *In Practice* 26:336–338.

Index

Note: Italicized page numbers refer to boxes, figures and tables